Intimacy AFTER BREAST CANCER

DEALING WITH YOUR BODY, RELATIONSHIPS AND SEX

GINA M. MAISANO

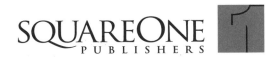

SQUAREONE
PUBLISHERS

EDITOR: Anna Comstock
COVER DESIGNER: Jeannie Tudor
TYPESETTER: Gary A. Rosenberg

Square One Publishers
115 Herricks Road
Garden City Park, NY 11040
(516) 535-2010 • (877) 900-BOOK
www.squareonepublishers.com

Library of Congress Cataloging-in-Publication Data
Maisano, Gina M.
  Intimacy after breast cancer : dealing with your body, relationships,
and sex / Gina M. Maisano.
     p. cm.
  Includes index.
  ISBN 978-0-7570-0324-0
  1. Breast—Cancer—Psychological aspects. 2. Intimacy (Psychology) I. Title.

  RC280.B8M2557 2010
  616.99'449--dc22
                              2010000497

Printed in Canada

10   9   8   7   6   5   4   3   2   1

Contents

This book is dedicated to every woman who has heard the words, "You have breast cancer."
You are so very beautiful.

Acknowledgments

After someone has fought cancer twice, their gratitude list becomes long. This book would not have been possible without the love and support I received from so many people, especially the wonderful women of No Surrender—my sisters and my dearest friends. What a chopper-ride it has been!

To the women and men who shared their stories with me and helped to round out this book so every view could be addressed, thank you for opening up such private parts of your lives so that others can benefit from them. The generosity of your hearts knows no bounds.

To all the men I have known who may find themselves, in one form or another, in these pages—no matter what happened between us, I think of experiences, both good and bad, as stepping stones to be learned from. I thank you for what I learned from each of you.

I must acknowledge, with deep respect and gratitude, every member of my medical team who has kept me in the winning column in the fight against the Beast since 2001: Marc Citron, Mansoor Beg, Lisa Berger, Alice Kim, Frank Tomao, Dominic Filardi, and everyone "up the hill," especially Charles Militana and Mervina Hinds.

In order to write this book I had to enlist the help of several experts in their fields. Namely Dr. Brian Cooperman, who saved my life so many times and who has always encouraged me, made me laugh, and taught me so very much; thank you for everything. Dr.

Ron Israeli, who has been unyielding in his kindness and support, generously shared his vast knowledge with me so I could pass it on in these pages; thank you. And Dr. Anthony Donatelli, whose incredible support and expertise helped make this book possible; I am grateful to you.

A special acknowledgment to Lilah Karpf—I learned a lot from you and it helped me with this book. Thank you for the time you spent with me. To Anna, for your infinite patience, brilliant editing, and warm encouragement, thank you so very much. And Rudy, you took a chance; you are a mensch and a friend, and I am forever grateful to you.

Without my family, I would not be where I am. I thank my mother for all that she taught me, because it helped in my life and in writing this book. And I thank my father, who has always supported and encouraged me; no matter what I did, he stood by me. My love also goes out to Joanne, Tom, Laura, John, Robert, and Sarah.

And finally, for David, this one's for you. We did it.

$\mathscr{P}$reface

I am the daughter of a beautiful woman. As a child, I would watch her get ready to go out with my father for the evening. She didn't spend a long time making up her face—she didn't have to. She would apply a little eye shadow, mascara, and powder, and then finish with lipstick. She'd emerge from her dressing area looking breathtakingly lovely. My clumsy fingers would help fasten her necklace or bracelet, and before I knew it, in a flurry of fur and the lingering scent of Cabochard, her cool cheek would press against mine as she kissed me goodbye and she would disappear into the night with my father for what always seemed like a magical destination.

I couldn't wait to grow up and be like her. I wanted to be as beautiful as she was. I wanted to have children and live in a pretty house like she did. And I wanted to find a man who was as strong, smart, and handsome as my dad was.

Things didn't exactly turn out that way, though. For starters, I worked. While I was busy building a business, my thirties caught up with me. It was getting a little late to find the life I had dreamed of. And then I was diagnosed with breast cancer for the first time. I quickly learned that my dream of children was now never to be realized. I saw my body endure a lumpectomy, radiation, and six months of chemotherapy. Nothing was turning out as I had expected. I found myself floundering and full of sadness.

Slowly I began to recover and I started to see myself as a woman again. I took chances and even fell in love. Like many breast cancer survivors, though, I wasn't as careful as I should have been. I fell in love with the wrong person because I somehow thought that I was damaged and couldn't do any better. The day I realized that I was settling for a bad situation because I thought I couldn't do any better, was the day that I reclaimed the self esteem I had before cancer and ended the love affair.

Not too long after that, I was diagnosed a second time with a different type of breast cancer. This meant that I would need not one, but both breasts removed. I had to decide what doctor to use and what type of breast reconstruction I would get in a hurry. Thankfully, I was blessed to find an artist who also practices as a reconstructive breast surgeon. Even though it was a bad situation, he made me absolutely beautiful.

I had nine months of chemotherapy and even more radiation the second time around, which unfortunately brought with it something the first cancer did not—sudden, horrible menopause, during which I experienced hot flashes and dramatic changes in my body. This chemotherapy-induced menopause turned out to only be temporary, but my oncologist put me right back into it medically to protect me from a cancer recurrence. In the two month respite I had from coming out of chemotherapy-induced menopause and then returning to medically-induced menopause, though, I went into action.

I made an appointment with my gynecologist. He is the man responsible for saving my life, because it was he who had insisted that I began getting screened for breast cancer at the age of thirty-five. Without that screening, my aggressive first cancer would not have been found until it was too late. He is also one of the most compassionate doctors a woman could ever have. I told him I could not handle the side effects that the loss of estrogen was causing, and he listened and taught me what to do. No other doctor had ever mentioned a rescue plan to me, and I was so grateful to him that I decided to spread the word to every other woman going through what I was. That became my life's mission.

I can now proudly say that I am the founder of a fast-growing, non-profit foundation for women with breast cancer. It helps them through every step of their disease, from diagnosis to life post-treatment. At the time, I wrote for a women's magazine geared toward women with breast and ovarian cancer. I contacted my editor there and told her that I wanted to write an article about bodily changes and sex after cancer. It took some convincing, but she agreed.

For the article, I interviewed wonderful women and doctors and found out all the ways we can reclaim our sexual selves after cancer—even in the throes of forced menopause. The article was a hit. It touched a nerve with many women who were feeling the same things I was, and they were hungry for more. I had been in contact with my publisher about another project, when I mentioned how important this topic was. I also had him read the article and told him about the responses I had received from women across the world. I felt compelled to write more on this subject. Thankfully, he gave me the go-ahead and thus, this book was born.

We *need* this book. As someone who has fought cancer not once, but twice, I believe in the future and making it the best it can possibly be. I live my life with hope and optimism. I don't shut myself off to the possibilities of the world just because I *had* cancer. On our foundation's website there is a support forum, and so many newly diagnosed women find us, scared and without hope. By the time the wonderful women of The No Surrender Breast Cancer Foundation are done with them, though, they are thriving. The very best part is that when many of them have completed their treatments, they turn around and encourage and coach the newly diagnosed women coming online just like they did months before.

That type of encouragement and hope is what I hope to accomplish with this book. Once you read it, pass it on to another woman who is living in a cancer frame of mind instead of living in the now. As someone who was once bald and bloated from steroids and had an extra eighteen pounds of chemo-weight, I know a few things about getting your body, hair, and skin back. I also know how important it is to lose that weight and get into shape. It can literally save your life by preventing recurrence. It is time we got it out in the open that, yes, there is life after cancer—a life that includes sexuality and love. And you do not have to suffer physically to accomplish that, either. You will learn how to slowly and comfortably change your body so you can enjoy lovemaking again.

While the relationships discussed in this book are between men and women, please do not think it does not apply to you if you are a survivor with a female partner. Most, if not all of the information will relate to you, as well. You also need to reclaim your inner goddess!

If you have just finished treatment and you still don't have any hair or eyelashes; if you have no desire for sex and feel like it isn't worth getting out of your sweatpants today, I am here to tell you, it is. My hair is long, I have great eyelashes, and I am in the best shape I have ever been. I have reclaimed my body, my confidence, and my desire, and I want to show you how you can, too.

It may take me a little longer to ever look as beautiful as my mom did, but I know how to make myself look as good as I feel, and that is the only thing that matters. I am happily single. Will I ever find "The One?" Probably. I'll know him when I meet him. But until then, I plan on kissing a lot of frogs, and loving every minute of it . . .

$\mathcal{I}$ntroduction

"Now, Voyager, sail thou forth,
to seek and find."
—WALT WHITMAN

More women are surviving breast cancer today than ever before, and not just until the statistical five-year benchmark. Many women are surviving for fifteen, twenty, thirty years and more. This is a testament to modern medicine. However, it does come with a price. While the medical community has been busy extending the lives of breast cancer patients, no one has been focusing on just what kind of lives these women are going to live.

Surviving cancer is not akin to finishing a book, closing it, and returning it to its shelf. With cancer, there is a web of continuing treatments and long-term physical and psychological side effects. There is also a never-ending fear that it will come back.

When you were first diagnosed you felt fine, but then your treatments began and they made you ill. In the blink of an eye, you went from being a woman to being a cancer patient. Now that your treatments have ended, you need to transition back into the land of the healthy and living. You must become a woman again and leave the cancer patient behind.

The artist Michelangelo believed that he didn't create his magnificent sculptures. He believed that they were always inside the marble blocks and all he did was uncover them. That is what you have to do. The beauty that is within you must be uncovered. It's time for the magnificent victor of the most frightening battle you've faced to emerge. But first you have to remove a lot of marble! You have to *want* to come out and be a part of the healthy world again. You have to believe that a beautiful life full of promise, opportunity, and love is out there waiting for you. When you do, the marble will melt away and you can begin to rediscover yourself and live beyond your cancer.

You have many exciting adventures ahead of you. Love and a fulfilling sexual life are attainable—they have not disappeared among the surgical scars, loss of hormones, and fear—you just need to be shown how to reclaim them. And you will.

If you are married, your husband's world was rocked by the news of your cancer. And now that your treatments are done, he may be wondering why you aren't bouncing back into your old routine right away. He wants his wife and lover back, but he is unclear about how the future will be for the two of you. A lot of changes have taken place in a relatively short span of time, and you probably aren't so sure either. Take a deep breath. This book will help you understand that through tender, open, loving communication, the two of you can rediscover your love life. You may even find it's better than it ever was!

Single survivor, your journey is completely different. Dating has never been easy, but breast cancer has now made it more complicated than you ever imagined. There is so much explaining to do, which is especially hard when you're vulnerable and unsure of how you feel about the new you. You literally need to fall in love with yourself and see just how beautiful you are before you can begin to fall in love with others and have them fall in love with you. You need to discover the strengths and features that make you desirable. Once you do, others will follow.

Daunting though it may appear, it's time for you—whether you're married or single—to start looking forward. Believe in yourself and all the beauty that you have inside. The first step toward your wonderful, new life is to divide and conquer. We need to break down what has happened to you medically and physically, and then find solutions to the long-term side effects you are left with. Part One discusses ways to counteract these side effects. Post-surgical challenges are also explained, and new ways of dealing with your new body are found.

Your psychological wounds will be dressed and stitched together, as well, so they can finally heal. Self esteem and body issues will be viewed in a realistic, open, and honest way—not in the way your doctor glosses over it, but in a way that will truly make a difference in your life. You will see that everything that has happened to your appearance has a solution. In fact, you may even end up looking better than you did before cancer!

After we accomplish your personal reclamation in Part One, we move on to your sexual reclamation in Part Two. Your treatments and medications have altered your hormones, which affects your sex life. But this book will teach you how to reverse adverse sexual conditions. If you are married, you will work out how to deal with your husband and family. If you are single, you will learn that your life is still ahead of you, and that your future can include both love and sex.

And speaking of sex, every question you have about your new, post-treatment body and how it will respond to sexual activity is answered. You will see that you can once again have a fulfilling sex life, and that your sexual future is exciting. Dating, love, intercourse, toys, and everything else your doctor didn't tell you is here in this book. Throughout these pages, you will also find personal stories that reflect real-world experiences of breast cancer survivors. You may find yourself in some of them. They are included to show you that you are not alone in any of this. There is a whole sisterhood right beside you feeling the same things you are, so take comfort in that.

Purchasing and reading this book means you are ready to make a change in your life. It means that you no longer want to be the "Designated Cancer Patient" in your world. Good for you girl! Your new life is waiting for you, so what are you waiting for? We've got work to do!

PART ONE

*Y*our Personal Reclamation

Hello, Survivor! You did it. You survived hearing the news that you had breast cancer and you learned everything there was to know about your disease in a matter of weeks. You are now fluent in doctor-speak and you can decipher a pathology report like a pro. You had your surgeries and you dealt with all the changes that came with the altering of your body. You even survived chemo. This has been some year.

Now your doctor tells you that you're done. Your calendar is strangely empty—no longer filled with treatment appointments and doctor follow-ups. Everyone congratulates you and thinks you will now magically return to the woman you once were. But they don't understand that woman is gone and a new one has taken her place. *You* may not even know it yet. Have you met the new you? She's in there. It's time to see who you have become and start living again . . . living the best life you ever have.

A lot of things are missing from the pretty pink catalog your doctor gave you when he first told you your diagnosis. You remember that catalog—the one with the picture of the pretty woman on the front, wearing a scarf around her head and bravely smiling into the camera. It glossed over your disease and treatments and let you know, in the briefest terms possible, that you would make it through

everything they were about to do to you. But they don't have a catalog for *after* they are done with you. They don't tell you about what
you are left with, and what you have to learn to live without, when
they send you home to live your life.

Your body has undergone a tremendous onslaught of chemicals,
surgeries, and even radioactivity. The doctors prepare you for it and
reassure you that your body will heal, but what about your spirit?
What about that inner resolve that got you up every morning, helped
you through each chemotherapy session, and kept you together
when you wanted to fall apart? Now that you have put down all
your weapons physically, it is time for you to heal emotionally. Only
when both your body and your spirit heal will you really feel like
you are "done" and can start living again.

In this first part of the book you will learn how to embrace the
new you, both physically and emotionally. You will learn how to fix
the things you can change and to accept the things you cannot. For
instance, you can't change how tall you are, so you must accept that.
But you can reverse the effects treatment had on your body, hair, and
skin, and you will discover, step by step, just how to make those
changes. Emotionally, you will learn how to live in the now. You will
learn how to look forward and maintain hope—not to look back and
worry about what could happen, because that is no way to spend the
rest of your life. You fought hard for your life, and that life is worth
living to the fullest. With some work and some healing you can make
your life better than ever, so let's get started!

1

$\mathcal{Y}$our Treatments Are Done. Now What?

You are finished with your breast cancer treatments, which is great! But they have undoubtedly left you with a host of collateral damages. Outwardly, your body has gone through many changes. You have had, at a minimum, one surgery—although you've most likely had closer to five once all was said and done. Additionally, you may have had radiation. The surgical side effects have almost certainly caused changes in your breasts, torso, and the arm on the affected side. If you had chemotherapy, you most likely lost your hair. You also gained weight, your skin is no longer the same, and if you weren't already in menopause, you are probably in it now.

This was quite a battle you waged and it shows. But the good news is that most of these adverse effects are not permanent. There are ways to aid and deal with healing, and in time, you can get back to your old self—maybe even become someone completely new who blows your old self away! Let's take a look at the various side effects you are facing, considering both those that don't go away, as well as the ones that do, eventually.

SHORT-TERM SIDE EFFECTS

There are certain unavoidable side effects that come with breast cancer treatment. Some only last for the short term, while others

7

can be permanent. It is important to remember that every problem has a solution. In most cases, the short-term effects solve themselves. Your hair will grow back, your immune system will improve, and as the last bits of chemicals leave your body, you will get stronger, look better, and feel like yourself again. There are some things you can do to speed up these processes, though, and they are as follows:

Hair Loss

Your hair will grow back on its own, *really*. And it will be as it was when you lost it. There are a few things you can do to assist its growth, though. For instance, the natural supplement Biotin will help your hair and nails get strong and grow again. Adding more protein to your diet in the form of eggs, lean meats, and dairy will also aid in your hair's recovery process. Over-the-counter baldness remedies, such as Minoxidil, have not been shown to help post-chemo hair growth; however, stimulating shampoos like Nioxin do help increase your scalp's circulation, and based on anecdotal evidence by breast cancer survivors, they help hair grow faster. There are no conclusive scientific studies to back this up yet, but it can't hurt to try. See page 41 for more information about hair care.

Neuropathy

Certain chemotherapy agents cause neuropathy, which is a numbness or pain in your fingers, hands, or feet. If you took any of the taxanes, including Taxol, Taxotere, or Abraxane, the neuropathy will take about three to six months to improve. However, taking vitamins B_6, B_{12}, folic acid, glucosamine, and chondroitin can help this process. There are also some medications that can help if your case is severe, but try the natural supplementation first and wait a couple of months before you ask your doctor for a prescription. This is because the drugs that are typically prescribed to treat neuropathy have side effects that can affect other parts of your life, as we will discuss later. If your neuropathy can be improved naturally, that will be your best choice in the long run.

Fatigue

You may find that you tire easily now, but in time you will get your energy back. During the healing process, don't be alarmed if you occasionally go from feeling wonderful to suddenly experiencing a chemo-crash flashback, leaving you exhausted like you felt during treatment. Although it sounds like an oxymoron, the best remedy for fatigue is exercise. Your energy levels will also improve if you eat a good diet, which means avoiding all processed foods including white flour, sugar, and junk food. Focus on eating nourishing foods that will stay with you and you should tire less often. That being said, don't hesitate to give yourself permission to take a rest if you are still experiencing fatigue. There is a lot going on inside your body as it recuperates, so let the process work itself out.

Chemo Brain

It's not you. Chemo really did mess with your brain. You did walk into the kitchen for something. . . . What it was, however, is anybody's guess. Rest assured, you are not losing your mind. The answer will come to you. As will that word you can't seem to remember—probably something difficult, like "bath mat." Studies have finally concluded what cancer survivors have claimed for years: They are foggy and forgetful after treatment. They can't remember names, forget what they needed at the market, have no clue when their mother-in-law's birthday is (well, at least now you have an excuse!), and so on. It will take you a good year before you are operating on all cylinders. The only thing to do in the meantime is to make lists. Then, remember where you left them.

LONG-TERM SIDE EFFECTS

In addition to the short-term side effects just discussed, chemotherapy has left you with some things you will always have to live with, or at the very least, be aware of. As with anything, however, early detection and treatment can sometimes reverse the changes that are taking over your body, so listen to it. You know your body better than anyone else. When it is telling you something, it whispers it first. Catch a problem in the whispering stage and it won't be a problem for much longer. But wait until it is screaming and you may be stuck with it. The following information discusses some of your treatments' more serious side effects so you can learn how to detect and deal with them.

Lymphedema

Of all of breast cancer's long-lasting side effects, nothing is more anger provoking and unfair than lymphedema, which is the swelling of the affected side's arm, hand, and even torso, due to the loss of one or all of the lymph nodes during surgery. Lymphedema occurs when protein-rich lymphatic fluid is unable to drain properly, and thus becomes trapped inside the skin's extra-cellular spaces. Since the lymphatic system works near the surface of the skin where the vessels are tiny, any scarring from surgery can affect the flow of the fluid and make it harder for it to circulate throughout your body.

Lymphedema is a serious medical condition. You must be aware of it because if you were to get an infection in, say, your arm, it could spread throughout your entire body and become very serious—even life threatening. Plus, the swelling it causes is not only horrible to look at, but it can sometimes become painful. Left untreated, you may begin to feel joint pain and mobility may be affected, which can lead to irreversible damage.

It's important to realize that lymphedema may not happen right away—it could strike as many as five years after your diagnosis and be triggered by something as simple as a mosquito bite. Regardless of when it surfaces, it is painful, disfiguring, and potentially life threatening. So, if you see your fingers, hand, or arm swell, get to a doctor right away and start treatment.

The Three Stages of Lymphedema

There are three stages of lymphedema. Learn them well so you will immediately know when you should get to the doctor. Your breast surgeon is the best choice, but any of your doctors can refer you to a good clinic that specializes in lymphedema treatment. The stages are as follows:

1. The first stage is the *pitting stage*, which means that when you press your thumb into the arm the indentation stays there for awhile before returning to normal. This is the ideal stage to catch lymphedema because with early treatment, you can still reverse it.

2. The second stage is the *spongy stage*, which means that instead of indenting, the skin on the arm will bounce right back when you press down on it. Additionally, this is the stage during which permanent hardening of the arm tissues can begin. It also means that fibrosis has begun. Fibrosis is scar tissue that has built up between the tiny blood vessels because they have been stretched so much by the swelling, and it may add to the pain you experience, as well. When lymphedema has reached the spongy stage, it is not always reversible.

3. The third stage is the *hard stage*, and it is the worst in which to catch lymphedema. During this stage, the skin neither indents nor bounces back when you press your thumb into it. Your arm is also very big, and the swelling is permanent and irreversible. Your joints may hurt and you may even have mobility problems.

As previously mentioned, listen and pay attention to your body. Do your best to catch lymphedema in its first stage. If you do, you will save yourself from a lot of problems and pain.

What to Look for and When to Look for It

You must take extra care to learn the difference between natural swelling, like the kind that occurs on a hot and humid day, and unnatural swelling, like the kind that is caused by lymphedema. Natural swelling goes down once you are inside and elevate your arm. Unnatural swelling does not—your arm will keep getting bigger with no relief, no matter how much you elevate and baby it. Another sign of unnatural swelling is when your arm begins to feel like plywood and is a paler color than your other arm.

If you feel that something is not right or you are concerned you are suffering from unnatural swelling, speak with your doctor as soon as possible. He or she can direct you to a lymphedema specialist who can help you stop the progression before it gets any worse. After all, the last thing you need is another permanent change in your life.

Treatment

The best treatment available for lymphedema is known as Complex Lymphedema Therapy. It is comprised of lymphatic drainage, compression bandaging, skin care, and physical therapy. This method creates new pathways for the lymphatic fluid, and also prevents it from becoming worse.

You will have to wear compression bandaging while in therapy, which can last from one week to one month. But it is a small price to pay for preventing a permanent disfiguring condition. And even though it may feel like another battle wound—another dreadful reminder of your cancer and all you have been through—this is one you can nip in the bud. The only time it is truly "bad" is if you ignore it and it gets to be too late to reverse or treat. Therefore, as soon as you recognize the symptoms, act immediately. You will be glad you did!

At-Home Lymphatic Massage

In addition to professional treatment, there is also an at-home massage technique you can use to improve lymphedema. It was created to redirect the drainage of your arm through the superficial blood vessels that are now doing the work of your missing lymph nodes. This do-it-yourself massage needs to be taught by a professional, but the following information will give you a quick idea of what it's all about. You *can* train your body to compensate with what it has available. It just takes time and patience.

The key to this massage is to wake up the other lymph nodes in your body and to get them to act as a siphon, pulling the fluid away from your affected arm. By massaging the lymph nodes under your collarbone, behind your shoulder, down by your waist, and in your groin, you can actually pull all the built up lymphatic fluid away from your arm and into your circulatory system where it can be flushed out. The massage of the arm goes in a downward motion towards your existing lymph nodes, making them do the job of your missing ones. Ask your doctor or lymphedema specialist to show you how to perform self-massage.

Prevention

To prevent lymphedema, you need to reduce the production of lymphatic fluid. Everything you do that increases blood flow to your arm or hand, such as lifting or scrubbing, also increases the lymphatic flow, so these and other strenuous, repetitive exercises should be avoided. You should also avoid extreme heat (hot baths, doing the dishes, etc.), exposure to the sun, and extreme cold. Additional items and activities that can trigger or worsen lymphedema include clothing that is tight around the affected wrist, tight bras that leave an indentation, carrying heavy bags with the affected arm, and getting your blood pressure tested on the affected arm. So, try to avoid these whenever possible. See the inset entitled "Lymphedema Triggers" (page 15) for even more things to be aware of concerning lymphedema.

Hormonal Hot Flashes

Chemo can have a profound effect on your hormones and may throw you into premature menopause. If your cancer was fueled by estrogen, your doctor may even opt to surgically induce menopause by removing your ovaries, or to chemically induce menopause by administering a monthly injection. With either of these occurrences comes a host of problems. But luckily, they all have solutions.

No matter what, all women will face hot flashes at some point in their lives. When you have had breast cancer, though, they may occur years earlier than they normally would have. And on top of that, you don't have the luxury of taking low-dose estrogen to counteract menopausal symptoms. This is because if your cancer was fueled by estrogen, the last thing you need to do is feed your body more estrogen. You shouldn't reach for plant-based hormones, either. There is quite a bit of scientific controversy surrounding phytoestrogens, which include soy and black cohosh. Since they mimic estrogen and reproduce the same effects of exogenous estrogens, you should probably stay away from them. You need to speak with your doctor about this.

So what *can* you do to alleviate hot-flash symptoms? First, let's talk about what items make hot flashes worse so you can do your best to avoid them. Coffee, tea, anything else with caffeine, alcohol, chocolate, spicy foods, hot tubs, saunas, and other things along those lines all intensify and increase hot flashes. Avoid them and reduce your hot flashes. Also, get your thyroid checked. Sometimes an incorrect dosage of a synthetic thyroid hormone, such as Synthroid, can make your hot flashes worse.

Exercise, dressing in layers, and avoiding the above-mentioned triggers will all help naturally alleviate your hot flashes. For night sweats, try keeping a fan that has a remote control in your bedroom. That way, should you wake up steaming, you can throw off your covers and turn on the fan without having to get out of bed; thereby enabling yourself to fall back to sleep faster. Also, use only natural fibers in your clothing and bedding—cotton breathes, polyester does not.

Vitamin E, Green Tea capsules, and B vitamins all help with hot flashes, as well. There are also a variety of medical options. Certain antidepressants can help, but be aware that SSRIs, which are a class of antidepressants, can also kill your libido. Additionally, there is a drug called Neuronton, which was originally created as an anti-convulsant medication and was later discovered to have the ability to deaden nerve pain in shingles patients. Since then it is sometimes given to help combat menopausal symptoms and lingering neuropathy. Like SSRIs, though, it decreases your libido and your ability to enjoy sex or reach orgasm. Finally, Donnatal, a form of phenobarbital that is normally given to people who have irritable bowel syndrome, has helped many women with hot flashes. Taken at night, it not only helps you sleep, but it can keep the night sweats away. Talk to your doctor about which options may be right for you.

Lymphedema Triggers

Even though there is never any guarantee that you won't get lymphedema, there are things you can avoid that will help prevent it from occurring. Take extra precautions with the following:

• *Shaving under the affected arm with a regular razor.* You have lost sensation under your arm, so you won't know if you have nicked yourself. Since your lymphatic drainage is compromised because of surgery, even the smallest nick while shaving can open the door for bacteria to enter your skin. Lymphatic fluid is a breeding ground for infection if there aren't enough channels for it to be filtered through your system. Therefore, make sure your razor is clean, new, and has not been sitting in a soap dish collecting bacteria, otherwise you will risk causing a serious infection that can become systemic.

• *Manicures and Pedicures.* Always bring your own tools to the salon, or make sure the tools they use on you have been sterilized in an autoclave that you can actually see—don't just take their word for it. Pass on cuticle cutting, as well, and instead have the manicurist simply push them back gently. If you are getting acrylic or UV Gel nails, make sure they are careful when they file down the nail beforehand. Tell them not to go too deep and to avoid the cuticle area with the power file. Ask if they can roughen the nail by hand with an emory board instead.

As with the shaving, a nick in your fingertip or nail can introduce bacteria into your skin. Your system is not able to clear itself of bacteria as well as it was before some of your lymph nodes were removed, because there are now fewer of them to filter the lymphatic fluid. Even a simple manicure can cause infection, so be aware of what to avoid in order to protect yourself.

• *Working in the garden.* Always wear gloves when you do yard work, because if you don't, you can easily scratch yourself and open your body up to infection. There are long, opera-length gardening gloves widely available that you should wear when tending roses or other plants you have to reach your arms into, in order to prevent cutting your skin.

• *Needle pricks, blood draws, and IVs in the affected arm.* Avoid having any needles stuck into your affected arm. Doctor's offices in particular have microbes, which can cause infections that your compromised lymphatic system cannot fight off naturally. If you have had bilateral lymph node removal and need surgery, speak to your anesthesiologist beforehand and ask that extra precaution be taken. For example, you might ask for the area to be thoroughly cleaned before the IV insertion with the same antibacterial solution they will use on the surgical site. Or, you might ask for a topical antibiotic to be put on the area where the needle enters the skin.

Additionally, tell your anesthesiologist that you can't be hooked up to the IV for too long after the surgery is over. The sooner it can be removed, the better. He or she should also take extra precaution and add a bag of IV antibiotics to protect you. If you require a very long surgery that will compromise your arm, request to have the IV put into your foot, instead. Speak to your doctor about your options. He or she will be able to offer the best advice for you.

• *Bug bites.* Always put on bug protection. Infections can not only be made worse by lymphedema, but they can also cause lymphedema. A simple mosquito bite can bring on a permanent change in your lymphedema status—from none, to full blown.

• *Animal scratches.* Keep Fido and Fluffy's nails trimmed. If you get scratched by your pet or someone else's, thoroughly clean the area and immediately apply a topical antibiotic cream. Every time your skin is opened by a scratch or a bite, bacteria enters your body. By immediately applying a topical antibiotic, you are helping your body fight an infection before it starts.

Picture a river that flows unimpeded. That is what a normal lymphatic system operating correctly is like. Now picture a stream with rocks and mud blocking the path of the water. It has some soupy puddles that are not flowing, but are stagnating. Without your lymph nodes, your lymphatic system transforms from the free-flowing river into the rocky stream.

The cleaner you keep your lymphatic fluid, the less chance you have that any "standing water" will breed bacteria and cause infection. The infection that can happen with lympedema is serious. It can spread throughout your entire body and sometimes require hospitalization. Only *you* can protect yourself, and the best way of doing that is by prevention. Keep alcohol wipes and antibacterial ointments with you at all times, and speak to your doctor about getting a prescription for oral antibiotics to have on hand just in case.

Low Libido

Having little to no desire for sex is both physical and psychological. Physically, it is no wonder you have no interest in sex, for all the reasons mentioned earlier. Emotionally, it is hard to get your mojo back because you have been through so much that you truly have a form of post-traumatic stress disorder. Take an inventory of all the medications you are on, including antidepressants, nerve-ending medicines, pain-killers, and others, as some of them can cause loss of libido. Then, try to switch to alternatives that do not have that side effect. The best antidepressant in terms of not causing the loss of libido is Wellbutrin. But as always, this is a discussion you and your doctor need to have.

Vaginal Atrophy

Without estrogen, your vaginal tissues can become thin and weak. They can dry out and as they attempt to heal, the tissue weeps a clear fluid. Unfortunately, this same fluid subsequently dries in a milky white film on the skin, making the area itchy and causing it to burn. This leads many women to believe that they have a yeast infection or a urinary tract infection when they don't. To prevent this from happening to you, keep the vaginal area moist at all times with any one of the variety of products that are discussed on page 86. Additionally, keep the blood flowing to the area at all times. Vaginal atrophy and the things you can do to reverse it are covered in more detail in chapter six (page 75). If you follow the exercises included there, you can reverse and end vaginal atrophy forever.

EMOTIONAL IMPACT

Physically, you are done with your treatments. But why don't you *feel* done? How can your doctor possibly say to you, "Okay, that's all folks!" when your battle with cancer really isn't over? In the matter of a few days, your life was changed forever by simply hearing that you had breast cancer. Then the horror seeped in as they told you all the things you must do to beat it. You toughened up and did them all. You put on your armor and fought each step of every battle. You won. But now you are exhausted. You are burnt out. You are so done with this. Why, then, when your doctor *says* you are finally done, are you so scared and vulnerable?

It's simple. You have to emotionally catch up to all that happened to you physically. And that takes time. Just as your body must heal, so, too, must your spirit. Emotional scarring is one of the hardest side effects to overcome, because after breast cancer you feel like you can never trust your body again. It's tempting to want to withdraw into yourself. However, if you do that it will only get harder and harder to climb out and find the help and hope that exists. Recognizing that you are not alone, that millions of women have felt, and are feeling, the exact same way you are, can help you climb out of your shell.

A big step in putting this whole "cancer thing" behind you is accepting that you did everything you possibly could to fight this Beast. You fought cancer and you won. The best revenge you can get is to make a conscious decision to change your living habits and live a healthier life. That is not to say you weren't living one before you were diagnosed, but there are studies that show that women who work out regularly after they've had cancer reduce their risk of recurrence by as much as 50 percent. Working out will also help lift your spirits and make you feel stronger and more confident.

Before cancer, you knew that you *should* make wise choices. After cancer, you know that making those same wise choices can save your life and your spirit. Once you start to take control of your life and you are no longer following orders blindly like a soldier landing on a beachhead, you can start to feel a distance between yourself and the horrors of breast cancer, and your spirit can now, finally, heal.

FEAR OF RELAPSE

Perhaps the most common question breast cancer survivors ask themselves is, "Will it come back?" They also wonder if it's even a question of *if*, or rather, a question of *when*. As you pack up your Christmas decorations are you thinking, "Will I be here to unpack these next year?" Are you watching your little daughters playing in the yard thinking, "Will I see them get married?" When you go to the doctor for a follow-up do your hands sweat and does your heart pound?

If you answered yes to any of these questions, the "Other Shoe Syndrome" has hit you. You got the first shoe when you were diagnosed, so you convince yourself that the "other shoe" must certainly be coming, and the fear of hearing those words again can be overwhelming. This fear is normal, and every woman who has been through what you have feels it to some degree or another—especially when she goes to the doctor because it is like returning to the scene of the crime. It was there that you found out your body betrayed you. But it was also there that you gathered up all that was necessary to get that body back in line. The next time you begin to panic on your way to a check-up, try focusing on those thoughts instead.

The hard truth is that yes, sometimes breast cancer can return. It can return as a new primary, which means that a brand new cancer appears in the opposite breast and you have to start from the beginning again. Or, it can return to a distant site, such as your bone or lung, which is classified as stage four metastatic disease. There really should be a stage five classification, though, because with all the advancments in treatment today there are millions of women living very full lives with stage four disease. They do all the things they did before cancer, only now they are monitored and need to be on some kind of treatment for the rest of their lives. Their lives are far from over, though.

Every early-stage cancer patient knows that reoccurrence is a possibility. However, it doesn't have to be a probability. There are things you can do to help yourself live a long, cancer-free life. Early detection in recurrent disease is just as important as early detection in primary disease, so don't skip those follow-up appointments. At the same time, though, don't live looking over your shoulder, waiting for another boulder to fall on you.

Look forward; move forward—always forward, never backward. Life cannot be lived in reverse. You can take the past and learn from your experiences, using them as stepping-stones to get through future situations, but always remember that your life is ahead of you. The most important day in your life is today. We spend so much time worrying about the future and regretting the past that we sometimes forget today is here. It is ours for the taking.

LIVE LIKE YOU ARE LIVING—NOT DYING

There is a country song where a cowboy sings about how his father, who is dying of cancer, teaches him to live like he is dying. People who don't have cancer often think this song gives great insight into living with the disease. Cancer patients, on the other hand, tend to think differently. What is the point of going through chemo and surgeries if you are going to spend your life like you are dying? What kind of life is that to live?

You are alive right now. Today, you are alive. And today is a good day because you can see the sunshine, smell the newly mown grass, and hear your children's laughter. That is living. Unfortunately, many women worry so much about relapsing or dying that they rob themselves of these simple joys. Is there a chance your cancer could come back? Yes. But if it does, do you want to be at the end of your life knowing you spent the last several years as someone who hid in the shadows and never went out, took risks, or celebrated life? Or, do you want to look back and see that you beat breast cancer, got back into living, followed through with plans, laughed, loved, and lived?

If you put things off, stop. Do them now. Don't postpone anything because of your cancer. When you live for today you don't focus so much on that other shoe, which is a very liberating feeling.

Emily, in Thornton Wilder's play, "Our Town," asks, "Life you are too beautiful to imagine! Do humans realize? Do they live every moment? Every, every moment?" To which the Stage Manager replies, "Poets and saints, maybe."

Be a poet. See the beauty around you. When you get overwhelmed, go outside and just *be*. Look at the grass grow and watch the clouds pass by overhead. There is so much more to you and your life than your cancer. Sometimes you need to step outside yourself to gain perspective. It is much better to live in the present no matter what may or may not happen to you in the future. Stop avoiding things because of what tomorrow may bring. You can't store your todays—they disappear—so live each one and make it worth remembering.

2

$\mathscr{P}$rescription and Natural Medications

ancer may be behind you, but you cannot escape the necessity of taking certain medications now and into the future. One of the reasons women are living so long after breast cancer these days is the addition of hormone, or endocrine, therapy treatments. These drugs combat cancers that need estrogen to grow, and also help prevent them from recurring. In addition, pain medication is sometimes required, and a course of antidepressants can help you adjust to life as a cancer-free civilian again, as well. In short, medications can help get your life back to normal and keep your cancer away. But, as with everything, good things sometimes come with a price.

HORMONE THERAPY

For the women whose breast cancers are estrogen and/or progesterone positive, drugs known as endocrine therapy can help them live a long, recurrence-free life. The oldest and most well-known endocrine therapy drug is Tamoxifen (Nolvadex). It is a selective estrogen-receptor modulator (SERM), meaning it blocks the action of estrogen in the breast and other tissues in the body where estrogen receptors hide inside cells. Pre- and post-menopausal women can take this drug to help keep their cancer at bay.

The second-generation endocrine therapy drugs are known as aromatase inhibitors (AIs), and include Arimidex (Anastrozole), Aromasin (Exemestane), and Femara (Letrozole.) They work differently in the body, and can only be taken by women who are post-menopausal. This is because their mechanism correlates with the way a post-menopausal woman's body synthesizes estrogen. AIs can help block the growth of estrogen-dependent tumors by lowering the amount of estrogen in the body.

Hormone therapy drugs are partly responsible for the lower mortality rate from breast cancer in recent years. They work. They keep your estrogen-dependent cancer away. However, they do have a down side. The side effects of these drugs can be debilitating. Women must work with their doctors to find a way to combat the side effects, which can range from joint pain, to GI disturbances, to loss of energy, to hot flashes, to general malaise. Additionally, your soft skin, your full, thick hair, your sexual desire, and your reproductive organs will all suffer, because they are also fed by estrogen.

However, there is solid proof that you will live longer and have much lower risk of a recurrence if you are on one of these drugs. So, take your medicine. There are large studies being conducted right now on patient compliance. It seems that some people stop taking their medicine at home because they do not like the side effects, because they start to feel better, or because they just don't want to take pills anymore. Don't let yourself be one of those people. If you have the opportunity to benefit from endocrine therapy, you have to find a way to stay on it and keep cancer away. It's essential for your well-being. Women who have estrogen- and progesterone- negative cancer don't have anything they can take after chemo. They *wish* they had the options and the hope that their estrogen-responsive cancer sisters have. *Take your medicine.*

ANTIDEPRESSANTS

You may very well need an antidepressant to get your brain chemicals working correctly again. So, when your oncologist asks you how you are feeling emotionally, be honest. If you are having a hard time dealing with life post-treatment, speak up. A short course of antidepressant medication can help enormously. However, it is important to note that some have sexual side effects and can decrease your libido. Be sure to tell your doctor you are aware of this, and discuss all of your different options with him or her so you can find the drug that is best for you. Please see page 170 for more information about depression and its warning signs.

PAIN MANAGEMENT

Some women experience lingering pain after their treatments are over. Others complain of ongoing pain from their hormonal therapy. The loss of estrogen alone can make you feel like the Tin Man on a rainy day. Many doctors will prescribe opioid pain medications to ease all-over pain. However, these should never be used as long-term drugs and they are not a solution to the pain problem. They are addictive and can only mask pain—not improve it. They can also make you loopy and cause you to lose your libido.

Opt for natural solutions to your pain whenever possible. For instance, if you have pain from your reconstruction, such as muscle tightness from your implants or expanders, try reaching for a muscle relaxant instead of a Vicodin. Non-narcotic relaxants don't zonk you out, and they actually treat muscle spasms and the pain that accompanies them, rather than only briefly making them subside. A good one is called Skelaxin and you should talk to your doctor about it. Additionally, pain from neuropathy can be helped naturally with vitamins B_6, B_{12}, and folic acid. And joint pain can be helped with glucosomine and chondrotin.

If your particular hormone therapy is causing you pain, wait it out if you can. Many of the side effects dissipate in three to four months. If they don't, switch to another type of drug. Pain from AIs can be reduced by making sure your vitamin D level is in the proper range. Go to your doctor to get it checked, and based on your results add supplements as necessary. If you are experiencing pain and inflammation from your surgeries, try taking a natural anti-inflammatory called Bromelain instead of an NSAID like Ibuprofin, which comes with side effects that can harm your stomach over long-term use. Bromelain is made from pineapple, and when taken with vitamin C, it can help you heal naturally.

Again, do what you can to avoid taking heavy-duty pain meds on a long-term basis. If you do take them, your quality of life will suffer because your head will be in la-la land and you will not be fully engaged in your daily activities. Your sex life will also suffer. Try some of the less harsh alternatives instead, and get out and exercise. You can do more for your body and reduce more pain with a simple walk or a swim than you think!

PERSONAL STORY:
HOW SWIMMING CHANGED MY LIFE

Swimming, quite literally, changed my life. I had lymphedema from my first breast cancer, during which I had a lumpectomy and had thirty-four lymph nodes removed. The lymphedema occurred out of the blue almost four years after my initial diagnosis, starting in my fingers before moving to my hand. Soon after, my entire arm was full and swollen. What was worse than the swelling, though, was the pain. My doctor sent me to a lymphedema clinic where I received a lymphatic massage and was then wrapped like a mummy from my fingertips to my armpit. This helped some, but it soon became evident that I was going to have to live like this forever.

Six years after my first diagnosis, I was diagnosed with cancer a second time in the opposite breast. One of my greatest fears was that I would get lymphedema in that arm, too. Sure enough, after a bilateral mastectomy and the removal of twenty-nine lymph nodes, I started to swell. I also developed infections in my arms because the fluid that was trapped couldn't be adequately filtered.

I went to a new clinic this time and started the same routine again—to no avail. There was no difference in my arm after the treatments, and now both of my arms were disfigured. They were an infuriating reminder of my cancer that I was forced to carry with me daily. But the disfiguration and the bulky bandages paled in comparison to the intrusive questions that were inevitably asked every time I went out in public. "What happened to your arms?" "Why do they look like that?" It was not funny and was none of anyone's business.

After my second round of chemo I decided I needed to get my body back in shape, despite my lymphedema. I had been a swimmer when I was young and I have always loved the water, so I joined the YMCA to swim and work out. As I approached the pool for the first time, I was worried about how it would feel to move my arms in the water due to my tissue expanders and bilateral lymphedema.

Much to my delight, however, it felt wonderful. I was weightless and able to glide through the water effortlessly. The scar tissue that had been causing me such pain in my reconstructed breasts broke up and I felt good again. My muscles soon appeared long and lean, and I built up my stamina. And then I noticed it. My hands looked normal again. My arms had definition again. The swelling was going down. The pool was saving me.

When I told my doctor about it, he informed me that movement through water is the best massage of all. The gentle pressure of being underwater helped to move the built-up fluid back through my lymphatic system and out of my arms. I felt great when I swam. I lost weight. My body looked better. And above all, I reversed my lymphedema. What an enjoyable way to rid myself of something so very ugly! To this day, I swim at least four days a week, twelve months a year. My gym membership to the Y was the best investment I ever made.

3

Taking Care
of Your Body

You will be amazed at what your body can do. Haven't you already been dazzled by its ability to fight the cancer beast? Sure, you are left with some after-effects, but they are nothing you can't conquer and this chapter will show you how. By overcoming what your treatment left you with, not only will you look and feel amazing, you will also reduce the chances that your cancer will come back. Not a bad deal, eh?

WEIGHT GAIN—CHEMO'S DIRTY LITTLE SECRET

One of the worst "jokes" about getting diagnosed with breast cancer is, "Well, at least I will lose weight!" This is nothing more than gallows humor, though, misguidedly believing that the chemo will make us lose those unwanted pounds. The joke is on us.

The reality is that women gain, not lose, weight during breast cancer treatment. The average weight gain from chemotherapy is between fifteen and thirty pounds. Additionally, according to a study done by Harvard Medical School Brigham & Women's Hospital, the more weight women gain post-diagnosis, the higher their chances of recurrence and death are. Researchers report that this finding is particularly high in pre-menopausal women who had a normal body mass index (BMI) before their diagnosis, and subsequently gained a sufficient amount of weight after treatment, raising their BMI's from "normal," to "overweight" or "obese."

So, TAKE OFF THOSE POUNDS NOW! There can't be better motivation to shed weight than knowing that women who maintained or lost weight after their breast cancer treatments had a lower risk of recurrence and death compared to their overweight counterparts. Now is the time to get fit and healthy. Here is how . . .

DIET

You really are what you eat. Remember that when you are making food choices. For instance, are you thinking about grabbing a high fat, greasy bit of junk food? Before you do, say to yourself, "I am what I eat," and then go for a lean, low-fat, healthy food instead. After all, wouldn't you rather be that?

Another trick to weight loss is to track what you eat every day. If you try to remember off the top of your head, you can conveniently forget certain items like the bag of Skittles you inhaled in the car. Therefore, keep an honest food diary and write down everything you consume, as you consume it. An honest food diary means *everything.* That includes cocktails and the small bites of food you steal off friends' plates. List the portion size, the time of day, and even what kind of mood you were in when you ate it.

Then, at the end of each day take a good look at what you put in your mouth. How much junk did you eat? Did you eat because you were sad or bored, or because you were truly hungry? How many servings of vegetables and fruits did you get in? This type of reflection is important because it will allow you to learn from your mistakes and make long-term improvements to your diet. And again, long-range studies have proven there is a direct link between diet and breast cancer recurrence.

According to the National Cancer Institute, "The Women's Interventional Nutritional Study, or 'WINS,' was the first large-scale randomized trial to show that a change in diet can improve breast cancer outcomes in women who are receiving conventional treatment for early-stage breast cancer." WINS proved that after five years, women

The Right Way to Eat

Healthy foods give you more nutrients, make your skin look better, and keep you living longer than their unhealthy counterparts, so why would you not make the switch from being a junk food junkie to a whole food goddess? The following chart shows you some easy substitutions you can make to immediately improve the quality of your diet. You'll then learn some tips that will really make a difference when it comes to the types of foods you choose to eat.

BAD FOODS VERSUS GOOD FOODS	
Bad	**Good**
White flour	Whole grains
Sugar	Fresh fruit
Hydrogenated fat	Olive, canola, and omega-3 rich fish oil
High sodium snacks	Fresh vegetables
Chemically processed foods	Lean proteins
Low fiber foods	High fiber foods
Fatty muscle meats	Nuts

Tips to Remember

- When shopping, read the labels and stick to the "Five" rule: Under five grams of fat, under five grams of sugar, and over five grams of fiber.

- Roast your foods slowly instead of sautéing or frying them. This brings out the flavor and eliminates the need to add extra fat.

- Switch from white rice to whole grain brown rice.

- Switch from regular pasta to whole grain pasta.

- Drink seltzer instead of processed sodas.

- Eat as few muscle meats as possible. All mammals are muscle meats. Try to restrict your intake to two or three times a week at a maximum.

- Choose organic milk, butter, and cheese to avoid consuming growth hormones.

- Increase your consumption of vegetables and fruits.

- If you can't pronounce the ingredients in a packaged food, do you really want to eat it?

- Margarine is just one molecule away from plastic.

Your pantry should resemble your closet after Labor Day and contain as little white as possible. White flour, sugar, and other processed foods all spike your insulin, which changes your metabolism and will cause you to store more fat. Those types of foods also clog your digestive system, which will keep toxins in your body for far too long. Additionally, healthier foods like olive oil are good for your complexion, and reducing your sodium intake will keep you less bloated and looking better. And the best part? Healthy foods taste better!

who decreased their fat intake by 24 grams per day had a 24 percent reduction in their relative risk of recurrence. What's more, women who were estrogen and progesterone receptor negative had a 42 percent risk reduction, which translates into an absolute relapse-free survival rate of 9.5 percent after 8 years.

So, how can you reduce your fat intake, and subsequently, your risk of recurrence? Read food labels. Check the fat content of everything you put in your mouth, including things you use to make your food tastier. For instance, a tablespoon of vegetable oil has 14 grams of fat in it. If you are attempting to stay within the WINS study guidelines of 30 grams of fat per day, things like this are important to note.

Take a look at your food diary and see where you can make trade-offs to mitigate your fat consumption. Consider switching from butter to olive oil or a light cooking spray. Buy a more expensive cut of meat that has less fat in it; the packaging should tell you how "lean" it is by giving you the fat percentage. Slow roast foods instead of sautéing or frying them; this brings out more flavor and virtually eliminates the need to add extra fat. Buy fresh foods and cook your own meals at home; this is the best way to control how much fat you are consuming per day. Restaurants use large amounts of fat because it makes the food taste better. And even when you think you're ordering healthy, you may not be. You may be shocked to learn that one of the fattiest menu items you can order in a restaurant is grilled vegetables. They are saturated in oil before they are grilled, and the vegetables used—zucchini, mushrooms, summer squash, etc.—are typically all very porous and absorb all the grease, making them higher in fat than, say, the menu's hamburger.

EXERCISE

You can't escape it. Exercise is important, necessary even, and it may very well keep you free from recurrence. A large-scale study out of Boston followed 3,000 women with breast cancer. It concluded that the women who did the equivalent of three to five hours of walking per week were 50 percent less likely to die from breast cancer, as compared to the inactive women. Both walking and more vigorous activity contributed to this benefit.

Similarly, according to the *Journal of the American Medical Association*, women who increase their activity level after diagnosis, whether or not they exercised before their diagnosis, increase their chances of surviving breast cancer. Women who participated in three hours of physical activity per week after treatment—for example walking for one hour, three times a week—cut their risk of breast cancer recurrence by 20 to 50 percent. The CDC recommends moderate intensity exercise for 30 minutes a day, five or more days a week. Women who follow this advice may survive longer than women who do not.

The take-home message is that once you are out of treatment, get back on track and start an exercise regimen that works for you. Design workouts that you enjoy and do them at least five times a week, for a minimum of thirty minutes each. To get in a good sweat you don't have to join a gym. Instead, you can walk your dog twice a day. You can play with your kids. You can become the best gardener on the block. You can mow your lawn and get a workout as well as a tan; not to mention how much money you will save on lawn-care service!

Start slowly, go at your own pace, and listen to your body to avoid injury. Every day, make sure you have done something active. Little things can add up to a lot. You might consider tracking your daily progress with a pedometer, as it is a great way to gauge how much or how little you moved. According to the National Institute of Health, your target should be 10,000 steps per day. It may take baby steps to get to your healthy goal, but they all count!

YOUR THYROID

If you received radiotherapy to treat your breast cancer, there is a good chance your thyroid was affected in some way. Start requesting thyroid tests with your regular blood tests at your oncology follow-up visits. If your thyroid is low, you will have trouble losing the chemo-weight, you will feel sluggish and depressed, and your hair will not grow back as fast as it normally would. A few months on a synthetic thyroid hormone such as Synthroid will make all the difference in the world, so be sure to have a thyroid discussion with your doctor.

VITAMIN D—THE FAT BUSTER

Studies have found that an overwhelming number of women diagnosed with breast cancer have a very low blood-level of vitamin D. Thus, increasing your vitamin D level now may very well prevent recurrence. Ask your oncologist to test your level. If it is low, he or she may start you on a loading dose of 50,000 IUs per week. After that, you can maintain your level with a fat-soluble capsule of between 2,000 and 3,000 IUs daily. You will soon discover that you have fewer body aches and pains, and that the adverse side effects from your hormone therapies are reduced. Additionally, you will find it much easier to lose weight. Add that to the bonus of possibly preventing breast cancer recurrence and you will wonder what you ever did without vitamin D!

DON'T FOLLOW THE SUN

Women who have had breast cancer are at an increased risk of getting skin cancer. Therefore, it is very important that you have a whole body skin check at least once a year. The sun has two types of rays, ultraviolet A (UVA) and ultraviolet B (UVB). Both of these damage your skin and can cause skin cancer. They are also the number one culprits in causing premature aging of the skin, wrinkles, discoloration, and reduced elasticity.

Even if you don't burn or have naturally darker skin, you are still at risk. The tanning process is your body's natural mechanism for protecting itself from the sun, and it happens no matter what shade you are. Also, it doesn't matter whether you are getting your tan outside or in a tanning booth, because both are harmful. In fact, tanning booths may be even more damaging than the sun, even though the owners of tanning salons like to claim they are safer. The truth is they concentrate the UVA and UVB rays so that they go deeper into the skin, thereby causing deeper damage.

Skin cancer can appear all over your body, but the most frequent locations are the head, face, ears, arms, shoulders, and neck. The lower legs are also susceptible. Now that you know the risks, it's important to learn the warning signs. If you suddenly notice that one of your moles has changed in size and appearance, go through this checklist:

- Has it gone from a round to an asymmetrical shape?

- Have the borders become rough and jagged looking?

- Did the color darken or bleach out?

- Has it started to bleed?

- Has it started to itch?

- Did the shape increase in size to larger than the diameter of a pencil eraser?

- Does it now rise up from the skin where once it was flat?

All of these could be signs of trouble. If you have a mole that you think fits one or all of them, it warrants a quick trip to the dermatologist's office. And, as with most health issues, the earlier you find skin cancer the easier it is to treat and cure, so don't wait. In the meantime, while you're outside wear sunscreen and keep reapplying it as often as it wears off. Wear a hat that shades your face, and if possible, stay inside between eleven and three, when the sun is strongest. Your skin will thank you and your prolonged youthful complexion will be your prize.

As a final note, if being pale bothers you and you do not want to walk around looking like Casper the Friendly Ghost, there are safe self-tanners and spray tan options for you. Several of them look great and don't age you or put you at risk for skin cancer. Just remember to apply sunscreen over the skin even after you are sporting your self-tan, because they do not protect you from the sun.

SMOKING

Even after some women undergo chemotherapy to rid themselves of breast cancer, they continue to smoke. They know that the survival rates for breast cancer are much higher than they are for lung cancer, but even that statistic isn't enough to make them stop. To a non-smoker, this whole concept seems insane. How can anyone take that risk? Wasn't breast cancer bad enough? The ugly truth is that it's hard to stop smoking. It is an addiction. But sister, if you are smoking, stop. Not tomorrow. Today. Right this minute.

If the horrors of getting lung cancer and having to undergo more chemo and more surgery don't scare you, maybe thinking about what it does to your appearance will. Smoking ages you more than any post-treatment medication, more than the loss of estrogen, and more than sun damage. It puts the aging process into overdrive, causing your skin to look not just years, but decades older than it is. You will get big, deep, non-repairable wrinkles around your lips and eyes, your skin will become blotchy and loose, and you will look as much as twenty years older than you really are—all because you smoke. So again, if the thought of getting lung cancer doesn't affect you, how about looking like an old lady before your time? Would that help you kick the habit?

Make yourself and your health a priority, and look into smoking-cessation programs. Your doctor can prescribe medications to help you over the initial shock of nicotine withdrawal, so quitting will become a little easier.

The bottom line is to be smart. Don't tempt fate. Don't beat one type of cancer only to get another, more deadly one. And remember your skin. Smokers' wrinkles don't go away, and the more they smoke, the deeper they get. And we're not even going to discuss a smoker's teeth and breath. We want you to be smokin' hot! If you're still smoking, you're not.

DRINKING

Alcohol adds empty calories and does not help you lose weight. This is because the sugar content in alcohol spikes your metabolism, which turns what you eat into fat instead of allowing your body to burn it off or turn it into muscle. Okay, so you know that already. But did you know that alcohol can bring your cancer back? Yes, it's true, and there are multiple studies to prove it. It doesn't matter if you are drinking wine or mojitos, either—alcohol is alcohol.

According to the Fred Hutchinson Cancer Center in Seattle, Washington, women who have two cocktails a day increase the chances of their breast cancer returning by almost 30 percent. The chance that it will be a more aggressive, invasive type of cancer is increased by 43 percent. Alcohol consumption is particularly dangerous in women who are post-menopausal. Since alcohol boosts estrogen production, it may diminish the effectiveness of their endocrine therapies in preventing a breast cancer recurrence.

Save your drinking for special occasions if you must drink. You can still go out with the girls for cocktails, but stick to those that are non-alcoholic. Cocktails even increase the chances of invasive breast cancer in women who have never had it before, so be a friend and encourage fun activities that don't revolve around martinis with your "civilian" friends.

FOR THOSE WHOSE CANCER HAS RETURNED

We've now talked a lot about how to prevent recurrence within the scope of taking care of ourselves. But what about women who have already had their diseases return? Where do they fit in? Right here. This book's focus is on *all* women who have undergone breast cancer treatments. Its purpose is to teach survivors how to get their lives back. Please, do not think that if your cancer has returned that the lessons we talk about do not apply to you, because they do.

If you are a woman with advanced disease, you now live with some type of treatment every day. You may or may not have lost your hair again, and you very well may be struggling with the sexual issues that come with being in treatment. But being a woman with advanced disease does not mean your life cannot be full of the excitement and joy that is expressed within these pages. While some of the suggestions may be difficult at best, you are still a woman, and you are still living, breathing, and very much a part of this life.

Celebrate each day you feel good and be aware that the same rules about enjoying life apply to you, too. If you are able to gain insight, hope, and some frisky ideas from this book, for the love of Heaven—go for it! Every bit of advice, every technique, and every encouragement to live the life you have now to the fullest, can and should be applied to the advanced-stage woman. Whether you were diagnosed at an advanced stage or you have progressed to one, you, too, can benefit from learning how to make a conscious effort to permit yourself to experience happiness and hope.

You are not a milk carton and you do not come with an expiration date. Your new treatments may be causing sexual side effects that are unacceptable to you. Be comforted in knowing that even in the middle of chemo, you can prevent and reverse the worst offenders of vaginal dryness and atrophy by following the techniques in chapter six (page 75). You, too, can begin to feel like *you* again.

The shock of a new diagnosis and the day-to-day dealings with cancer can put a damper on your libido. Get ideas here, and then speak to your oncologist about which are allowed and which are not. If you can switch your antidepressant to one that won't rob you of your sex drive, try it! If pain is getting in the way of enjoying life, get a pain management specialist to help you. Once you have identified the problem, you can begin working to correct it.

You have experienced what every early-stage woman is afraid of: You heard that your cancer returned. However, you also learned that just because it returned, it didn't mean your life stopped. It just meant your life became more of a challenge. You now have to take treatment again, and your goal has changed to achieving stability in your disease. Never, though, did you stop being a woman. Having metastatic disease does not mean happiness and love are no longer allowed in your life. It simply means you have to reach a little bit farther for them. Find the hope and joy that is still around you and appreciate every second of it.

To all women with advanced disease, this book also applies to you. We are all sisters in this disease, and no one, regardless of her situation, is discounted or left out. While you are reading, remember to include yourself in every plan, technique, and exercise, because your life is not over—not by a long shot.

4

$\mathcal{I}$mage Reconstruction

I sn't it about time you stopped standing by and letting things happen *to* you? You are done with your cancer and your treatment, so now is the time to start making things happen *for* you. When you were first diagnosed and throughout your treatment, you were constantly told what to do, what not to do, and everything in between. With so many people pulling your strings, it was undoubtedly hard to be a confident, self-reliant woman.

That is all behind you now. This is *your* time and you want to look your best. Taking extra time to be gentle with your skin and hair can make all the difference in the world when it comes to your appearance. On the other hand, the previous chapter taught us that smoking and drinking are beauty zappers. You have several repairs to make after chemotherapy's chemical assault. With that in mind, our discussion starts at the top with ways to care for your hair, and then moves on to products and procedures that can improve the look of your skin.

YOUR HAIR

There is no getting around it. Losing your hair during treatment is almost as hard as hearing you had cancer in the first place. You get used to it, but you still dream about it. Your hands still reach up to push a loose lock from your face long after all the locks have gone.

When it *finally* starts to grow back, it is like a miracle. First you see peach fuzz. There is really no color to it, but there is definitely something happening up there. Then the short sprouts make their appearance, and before you know it, you are measuring how long it has grown every week.

As exciting as that can be, the hair that comes in is not like the hair you lost. The color, texture, and consistency are all different. It may be totally grey or jet black where it once was blonde. It may be dry and coarse where it once was healthy and fine. And most commonly—it is curly. It takes about two years for your hair's original consistency to return. But each day you see the new growth come back should be a celebration, because it represents another step away from cancer. The sooner you can ditch the wig or scarves and go "topless," the better you will feel, because it somewhat symbolically marks a line between being sick and not being sick anymore. So, here are some tips to get that hair growing and to help you look your best:

Supplements

Start taking Biotin—a vitamin supplement that helps with hair and nail growth. Ask your doctor before you start any supplement, but Biotin is harmless and it really does help. One tablet of at least 500 mg a day is a good start. Biotin is also found naturally in eggs, nuts, and avocados, so try adding some to your diet.

Stimulating Shampoos

There are special shampoos that stimulate blood flow to the scalp, so use them! The most popular is Nioxin. Buy the one for thinning, fine hair to work on hair re-growth. Nioxin also offers a stimulating serum. Be careful with this item, though, because your scalp is sensitive after chemo and this serum may be too rough on you. It's a good idea to massage your scalp, as well. Doing so will increase blood flow and wake up your hair follicles.

In addition to Nioxin, there is a Rogaine (or minoxidil) for women. However, the jury is still out on whether it helps at all with hair re-growth after chemotherapy. This is a question for your doctor—preferably a dermatologist who deals with both hair loss and skin.

Finally, note that it may not be necessary to wash your hair every day. Doing so can dry it out. If your hair looks terrible in the morning, simply rinse it under the shower and only apply conditioner—skip the shampoo. This will save your hair from being stripped of its natural oils and you protect it from further damage.

Styling Products

One thing all women agree on is that hair, post-chemo, is on curl overdrive. In the beginning you get a Brillo Pad look, which eventually grows into all-over bouncy curls like Shirley Temple had. Rest assured, they can be tamed with a little effort. First, make sure your hair is conditioned. Use a good conditioner that will moisturize and protect your hair from any heat appliances you may use. You should also buy a control pomade, a spiking gel, a frizz tamer, a spray-on conditioner, and a good flat iron. After shampooing and conditioning in the shower, apply the spray-on conditioner. From there, you can smooth back or spike up your hair with the gel.

If your curls are still so frizzy that you look like a Chia Pet, then apply some of the anti-frizz serum. If that doesn't help, a mini flat iron can smooth out the hair. You need to purchase one that is small, about a half-inch wide, because your hair is too short for a normal-sized one. Still, even with the smaller size, be very careful not to burn your scalp. You have to be careful not to burn out your new hair, too, so use your flat iron sparingly and always apply a heat-protective product first. Use trial and error to figure out which products and styling techniques work best for you.

Professional Help

If you really want a boost and you want your hair to look not only smooth and shiny, but *longer*, too, invest in a salon treatment. For about $200 or more, you can get a Keratin straightening treatment. The stylist applies a Keratin-based product to the hair, dries it, and then flat irons it perfectly straight. The Keratin seals the hair, makes it softer, and tames the curls. You can't wash it for 72 hours after the treatment, and you can't use clips or elastic bands during that time or your hair will take the shape of them. After you eventually wash your hair, though, you will see that the corkscrews are gone. The frizz is also history. And the best part, because it is so soft and straight, your hair *looks longer*. These treatments, while expensive, last three to four months and really help get you over the hump of being a "Brillo head." Please note that you will have to use a special, phosphate-free shampoo if you get this treatment, because phosphates remove Keratin. They are sold everywhere; if you check labels, you'll find one.

There has been some controversy surrounding formaldehyde-made Keratin treatments, because some believe it is a carcinogenic. That's just what you need—cancer-causing hair treatments for hair that is growing in from cancer treatment! Be sure you shop around. There are formaldehyde-free Keratin treatments, as well as some that have a very low percentage of it. You should not use anything with more than 2 percent formaldehyde. The risk of anything happening to you is actually extremely low, but there is a danger for the salon specialists because they breathe in the fumes when they are flat ironing your hair. Always take an extra precaution anyway, and ask for a towel to hold over your mouth and nose during this part of the treatment to avoid breathing in any of the fumes. Also, request to have a fan blowing near you or to be seated in an area with adequate ventilation.

Color

Color is another wonder after your hair begins growing in again. Battleship grey, translucent, and snow white are all some of the surprise new colors you may see. Or, if you colored your hair for several years before your diagnosis, you may finally see what your natural color was for the first time in a long time.

Hair "takes" color differently after treatment, so it is best to go with a professional the first time. You may only need highlights to get you through the initial growing stages if there is not enough hair to color. Your colorist will know best. If you end up doing it yourself, you may not be happy with the outcome so don't throw out your wig just yet!

Eyelashes

Your eyelashes may have fallen out a few times during your treatment. This is common, especially if you took Taxol, Taxotere, or Abraxane. Then, just when you think they have all grown back, you see them coming off again. Eventually they will stay, but if they do not grow back as full as they once were, ask your dermatologist or reconstructive surgeon about the prescription drug called Latisse. It was originally invented for people with glaucoma. After using it, patients noticed that their lashes had become thick and dark, so now it is also used specifically for eyelash growth. It is applied with a brush across your lid—similar to the way liquid eyeliner is applied—before you go to bed each night, and it really works. It will make a significant difference in your eyelashes in as little as two months.

With that being said, it is important to know that Latisse can lower your eye pressure. To prevent this from happening, you must be very careful not to get *any* product in your eyes. Be sure to have regular check-ups with your eye doctor to test your pressure, as well.

YOUR SKIN

Not only is your hair affected by cancer treatment, your skin changes, too. The chemical assault from chemotherapy, not to mention the stress you were under during it, shows up in your skin. It lost some elasticity, your pores seem to have grown and multiplied, there are a few more lines where there weren't any before, and you may find the dreaded "Chemo 11" in the mirror looking back at you; you never had a mark on your brow bone before, but now you are branded with the number eleven right smack dab between your eyes.

A lot of this has to do with the hormonal changes you went through. Chemo turns off your estrogen, which is one of the hormones that helps keep your skin looking young. It is also dehydrating, and that shows up, too. Now that treatment is over, it's time to take care of your skin. Most of it you can do at home, but for some of it you may have to call in the professionals.

Cleansers

First, evaluate your current skin-care routine. What kind of soap or cleanser are you using? If you must use soap, the only brand of mass-marketed, commercial soap that you should use on your face is Dove. Every cosmetic expert and dermatologist agrees on this. All of the other brands are too harsh and strip off too many of the natural oils you need. Natural-based soaps are always a better option. They are a bit more costly and don't last as long, but if you find a good olive-oil-based soap and can fit it into your budget, go with it.

If you use a liquid cleanser made for faces, look at the ingredients and make sure it does not contain harsh chemicals. Your skin is not as tough as you may think, and as you age, it becomes thinner and more fragile. What you do now can make you look younger later, so take some time to reevaluate your skin post-treatment to see if your old cleanser still applies. You may find, for instance, that you no longer have oily skin and now need to make the switch to a cleanser for dry skin.

As a rule, less is more when it comes to cleansing your skin on a daily basis. Every night you should remove all your makeup with an appropriate cleanser for your skin type, and then apply your evening moisturizer. In the morning, you simply need to rinse your face. There is no need for heavy cleansing since all you are removing is moisture. Dab your face dry, apply your daytime moisturizer and daytime eye cream, and then proceed with your makeup application.

Exfoliators and Peels

Dead skin can make your complexion look drab and lifeless. You need to exfoliate. Do not, however, be tempted to buy products with ground cement and pebbles in them—you need to exfoliate, not strip the paint off the side of a house. Use a gentle exfoliator made from fine particles, not big chunks, three times a week. You do not want to overdo it, because if you do your pores will look larger and your skin will look worse.

In addition to exfoliators, another way to clear off dead skin is with do-it-yourself peels. (More on professional peels later.) There are some very good over-the-counter peels you can use. Look for the ones that have Glycol or Glycolic Acid high up in the list of ingredients. These peels come in kits or as masks, and you should follow the package instructions carefully. Generally, you want to use them about twice a week, but don't use them on the same day you exfoliate or you could irritate your skin.

Moisturizers

Moisturizing your face and neck after cleansing, exfoliating, and peeling is very important. Your neck can show signs of aging long before your face does, so don't neglect to apply moisturizer to it every time you apply it to your face. You also shouldn't neglect your eye area. The skin around your eyes is very sensitive, so when you moisturize, be sure to also apply a specially-formulated eye cream lightly with your little finger, so as to avoid using too much pressure.

When shopping for a moisturizer, it is important to remember that just because something costs $300 does not mean it works better than something that costs $20. The ingredients are what are most important. There are wonderful products out there that have every ingredient combination imaginable. Some of these ingredients are complex and hard to pronounce, so learn how to be an expert at reading labels before you go looking. Know your ingredients. An educated consumer can make the best purchase of the best product that offers the best results for her skin.

A quick note about label reading: When products list ingredients, the ones that are listed first are the ones that are highest in concentration and amount. So, if you see Glycol, for example, as the last ingredient after fragrance, then it is a miniscule amount and it won't help you. When buying moisturizers, try to find one that has the following ingredients in its top ten:

Alpha-hydroxy acids

Alpha-hydroxy acids—including glycolic, lactic, tartaric, and citric acids—help decrease age spots or discolorations, reduce pore size, and help with fine lines. Look for a product with at least a 10 percent concentration. It may cause redness and slight irritation at first, so only use it every other day until your face adjusts. Then, slowly work up to everyday use. Also, be very careful in the sun when using a product that contains alpha-hydroxy acids.

Beta-hydroxy acid

This is also known as Salicylic acid. You remember Salicylic acid. It was in the Clearasil you used when you were a teenager. The good news is that in addition to acne, it also works on wrinkles, rough skin texture, and discoloration, which can all occur post-treatment. It is an exfoliant, too, so it removes the dead layers of skin, revealing the new and improved skin underneath. If your skin is very sensitive and cannot tolerate alpha-hydroxy acids, Salicylic acid may be a better choice for you. Studies have shown that it is less irritating and just as effective.

"King" retinol

This is the good stuff that is made from vitamin A. Retinol dives down to the lower layers of your skin where your collagen and elastin live. It stimulates them and helps to rebuild your skin from the inside out. It improves texture, pore size, wrinkles, and color, and helps return moisture to skin. You can get a prescription strength Retin-A from your doctor. Or, if you travel outside the United States, many of the prescription-only formulations of Retin-A are available over the counter.

If your skin is sensitive or not ready for the full-court press of prescription strength Retin-A, retinol is the next best thing. This brings us back to package inspection and label reading. Some over-the-counter formulas say they have "retinol" in them. But make sure that is exactly what you read. If you see "retinyl palmitate" instead of "retinol," know that it is a weaker version and you may not get the same results. In other words, don't waste your money. Look for a product with the actual "retinol" you want.

L-ascorbic acid

This is better known as vitamin C. It is proven to stimulate collagen, which is important because your body does not produce as much after chemo and chemo-pause. Get your vitamin C, both topically and internally, and reduce wrinkles, fine lines, and even scarring. When looking for vitamin C on a label, only look for L-ascorbic acid. Things such as magnesium ascorbyl phosphate, ascorbyl palmitate, and more, are not what you want, because they do not work as effectively.

Hyaluronic acid

Hyaluronic acid holds more moisture in the skin than any other substance, keeping it supple. When used in combination with the other skin care products, it makes for a complete treatment. Hyaluronic acid is found in your body naturally in the connective tissues. But aging, smoking, and chemo can all destroy your levels of it. Use a product with hyaluronic acid in it regularly, and watch the "Chemo 11" go away.

Copper peptide

Copper peptide helps promote the body's ability to produce hyaluronic acid. It helps to rebuild collagen and elastin, and to strengthen and rebuild the skin. It also makes skin firmer and tighter, and rids it of damaged collagen and scars.

Alpha-lipoic acid

Where the other antioxidants help correct past damage, alpha-lipoic acid helps prevent future damage. It improves skin's texture, color, and fine lines, and increases the effectiveness of vitamin C and alpha-hydroxy acids.

Soy

Soy is a plant as well as a phytoestrogen, which mimics women's naturally occurring estrogen. Skin care products that contain soy are said to reverse the signs of aging, because soy brings the missing estrogen back to the skin. It is also reported to decrease lines and wrinkles, and help tighten sagging skin. But here's the rub . . . does it get absorbed systemically?

No one knows the answer to that. If your cancer was responsive to estrogen and you are taking medication to turn off the estrogen in your body, do you want to take the risk of adding estrogen through your skin care? Keep in mind that soy is a plant estrogen and no one knows definitively whether, or how, it affects women with hormone-dependent cancer. Regardless, you need to speak with your oncologist and decide whether it is a risk worth taking.

Natural Oils

Olive oil, especially the extra virgin variety, reduces sun damage when it's used on the skin. It is a completely natural substance that just happens to moisturize wonderfully! You can use it anywhere on your body, including your hair. After shampooing, rub a little in your hands and run them through your hair, particularly at the ends. Also, the next time you take a bath, add a couple of drops of olive oil—or almond oil, which has almost no odor—and soak in it. Put the water on your face and let the oil penetrate. When you come out, you will be glowing.

PLASTIC SURGERY

Some wrinkles don't go away. Sometimes the "Chemo 11" is a permanent brand, and some pores are so hopelessly large and ungainly that no amount of at-home tending can reduce them. But, you know your reconstructive surgeon? Guess what else he does? *Plastics*. The next time you are at his office getting your reconstruction checked, ask about what other things can be done. If you feel you want to look better than ever, there are several ways to get you there. And your plastic surgeon has all the tools.

Botox

All those perfect looking thirty-something starlets know the secret to Botox: Use it while you're young. If you start early enough on the baby wrinkles that are just beginning to form, then they won't ever be able to grow up to be big, deep wrinkles. This is because Botox will have smoothed out the skin. You don't have to be a starlet to use it for this purpose—the same applies for you! You can stop the progression of the "Chemo 11" with a little hit of Botox now, before it gets any deeper.

Botox is made from botulitum toxin type A, and is a non-surgical, injectable treatment that reduces the contractions of the muscles that cause frown lines—a.k.a. the "Chemo 11"—that have developed. Plainly speaking, it paralyzes the muscles that are contracting, thereby relaxing them and making the surface of your skin smooth and soft. The wrinkles either melt away altogether, or become very faint.

With a good doctor, you can get a little Botox here and there that will stop wrinkles by targeting the muscles that are causing the most trouble. These are typically between the eyes, brow, and crow's feet. A doctor that starts small, with an easy touch, can make you look completely natural—not have the look like you are in a state of shock or a face so frozen you cannot make any facial expressions. Botox can and should be done subtly, as something to relax your furrowed brow and get rid of your wrinkles in a few key areas. In the long term, it will help keep them from growing deeper.

Botox injections are not painless, but you can numb the area first with an ice pack. Even though the needles are small, they burn a little, but the pain goes away in a couple of minutes. After your injections, you should not lie down for a few hours, nor should you rub the newly injected area. You may also get a slight headache, but it passes.

You won't see the full results of your Botox for two weeks. It is then that you should go back and see your doctor to see if you require some tweaking here and there. The results last for four months or so. When you start to notice that your forehead moves more, it is a sign that the Botox is wearing off and you should make another appointment with your doctor.

As with most things, Botox carries some risks of results that are not ideal. If your doctor has a heavy hand or if you have a heavy brow, your forehead muscles can become so lax that the skin of your brow will begin sagging down onto your eyelids. This effect is at its worst for about three weeks before it slowly dissipates. If this is a problem for you, it may mean that your forehead needs a lift. A good doctor will examine you and evaluate your brow and forehead before the injections. If there is a question about how it may affect you, the doctor may opt to avoid injecting the muscles higher up on your forehead and just concentrate on the lines between your eyes.

Cosmetic Injectable Fillers

But wait, there's more! Your doctor's bag of tricks includes more than just Botox, so don't think that is the only choice you have before a full-blown face lift. Most aging in the face is caused by a loss of volume. This is where fills come in. Radiesse, Restalyne, or Juvaderm can be injected into the lines around your mouth, which will plump up your skin and fill out your face. If you are in the early stages of the aging process, this can look like an instant and much cheaper facelift. It costs about one quarter of the price of a lift and can be done in a matter of minutes at your doctor's office.

If you opt for Botox first but still have some wrinkles, your doctor can put in a filler. Think of it as caulk injected into the skin just under the wrinkle that will plump it out so it disappears. Even your own fat can be harvested from your butt or abdomen and injected into your wrinkles. This can be a good option because you won't get a reaction from your own tissue, but it is not so great if your body reabsorbs it. Follow the advice of your doctor.

Most fillers stay for six months to a year. Some break down and create collagen production, which then fills out the wrinkle in place of the filler. These fillers are commonly used for the lines around the mouth, the lines from the mouth to the chin, and sometimes for filling out the cheeks.

Again, it is best to start slowly and conservatively. You also want an experienced doctor performing this procedure, because the results are not necessarily dependant on the filler you use, but on the Filler who is injecting it. Getting fills hurts more than Botox injections, because the needle is larger. You should definitely ice the areas of your face beforehand, or use a numbing cream an hour before the appointment. Your doctor may also use some lidocaine to help with the pain.

Your face will be swollen afterwards, and it will hurt, too. If you are on any blood thinning medications like Plavix, or if you take vitamin E or non-steroidal anti-inflammatory drugs like Advil or Alleve, you will bruise. It is best to stop taking these medications at least a week before the procedure, but check with your doctor before you do. If the bruising is bad, use make-up to cover it. But don't use make-up the day of the procedure, because you want to keep the area clean. You can also purchase over-the-counter Arnica gel, which can be found in health food stores, and apply it to the bruised area. This speeds up healing. As the weeks go by, you will see more and more improvement. But you should still see your doctor for a two-week follow-up to make sure you are even and no tweaking is necessary.

Chemical Peels

There are peels and then there are *peels*. The mechanism of a chemical peel is to smooth the skin by removing its damaged outer layers. Your doctor has the good stuff that can literally lift away years of skin damage from sun exposure. If you are considering a chemical peel, there are three main types that use three different chemicals, including alpha-hydroxy acids, trichloroacetic acid (TCA), and Phenol.

The least abrasive peel is made from alpha-hydroxy acids (AHAs). This is usually a glycolic peel. You can buy glycolic peels over the counter, but your doctor has them in stronger concentrations. The next level up is a weekly version of the glycolic peel. Once the desired result is obtained, daily maintenance can be done at home with creams and cleansers. There is virtually no recovery time from a glycolic peel, but you will leave the office with red skin. Additionally, your skin may become irritated and will sting little. It will also crust over before it sloughs off to reveal the new, brighter skin underneath.

If you want to go even deeper, your doctor also has trichloroacetic acid (TCA) peels. These can reduce the appearance of rough skin texture, fine wrinkles, and the pigmentation problems associated with sun damage. They can be used in many concentrations, but are most commonly used for medium-depth peeling. TCA peels cause the same redness and burning as the AHA peels, but you will also be very swollen and the subsequent crusting is significant. A TCA peel can change the color of your skin, as well. You absolutely must avoid the sun for at least six months after getting this peel, because your new skin is very delicate and vulnerable. You may need to go more than once for a desired result.

If you have skin that needs even more work yet, your doctor has one more level up: the Phenol peel. The Phenol peel is the ultimate peel. It attacks deeper wrinkles and damaged skin pigmentation from over exposure to the sun. It can even remove pre-cancerous growths. Phenol bleaches the skin, so it is not advisable for use if you are a woman with a dark complexion; the skin on your neck is too delicate. If you use it, you will have the undesirable result of a light face and a dark neck.

Recovery from a Phenol peel is long, and it may take months before you can see the final result. Your face will swell after the peel, and in some cases, your eyes may be swollen shut. You will be on pain medication and you should not talk or chew for the first few days—a liquid diet is recommended. You will need help at home after this peel. It is a big deal and you need to be prepared for it. The recovery is almost as intense as it is for a facelift. The only difference is that there is no surgery involved.

Facelifts

Are you there yet? Do you really think you need one? Do you really think you want one? If your answers to these questions are "yes," it's time you have an honest, heart-to-heart with your doctor. If he or she doesn't do faces, go to one who does. You may just need certain areas done, so be sure to discuss all of your different options.

An eyelift will remove the extra skin that makes your eyebrow heavy and weighs down your upper lid. The surgeon clips off the excess skin and hides the scar in the crease of your lid. This procedure really opens your eyes again. If you have bags under your eyes, they can remove fat and extra skin and tighten that area up, too. A forehead lift can be done with small incisions under the hairline, through which a surgeon separates the muscle from the bone and pulls it up. Excess skin is then trimmed. This makes your face more open and less tired or angry looking.

Additionally, there are partial facelifts. These lift the muscle by the outer cheekbone and pull up that section of your face so you no longer have those deep lines, known as marionette lines, around your mouth. The scar is usually by the ear. And finally, a full lift takes care of all these areas, as well as the jowls and neck. It is really important to have a good doctor who respects the integrity of your facial structure. Everyone knows what a bad facelift looks like, and you don't want that. The good ones are undetectable, because the patient looks rested, refreshed, younger, and as a result, very, very happy!

A note about nice doctors: Sometimes having a super-nice doctor can be frustrating. If you ask the plastic surgeon who did your reconstruction about some "freshening" you may want done on your face and he looks at you, smiles, and says, "You look fine!" that is lovely. But that is his opinion. Don't just turn away and say, "Oh, okay, never mind." Talk to him. Tell him that you see a change in your face and point out the specific areas that are bothering you. When he sees you are serious and not just looking for reassurance, he will take another look and give you his opinion and hopefully, your options.

THE BOTTOM LINE

You had a long, emotional, and exhausting battle. If it is showing up in your face or your hair and you don't like it, there are things you can do to fix it. Some women may choose not to do anything because they are plum worn out. But, some women choose to take one or more of the steps just discussed because they represent reclaiming their lives. Making yourself pretty is a positive move. Feeling good about who you are and what you look like is such a treat after having felt so very dreadful for so long. It is up to you. How do you want to look? If you are happy with your current self, that's great; but if you want to make some improvements, don't be afraid to go for it . . . be as beautiful as you can be!

5

$\mathcal{G}$etting to Know the New Girls

No matter what kind of surgery you had, you undoubtedly experienced a sense of loss; it's an emotional experience to have someone cut into your body. No surgery is easy, either, so don't let anyone minimize your experience. Many women who get lumpectomies often get comments from ignorant people who say that they must not have had a "bad cancer" because they still have their breasts. This is hogwash. All cancer is bad whether it is confined to your ducts or spread to distant sites.

Your privacy was already invaded by cancer and doctors, and now it's being prodded by friends and family members who want to know why you made the decisions you did to rid your body of the cancer. Remember that not everyone is as well informed about breast cancer as you are, so sometimes they can say stupid things. When that happens, do your best to politely ignore their comments and judgments, and just focus on doing what's best for you.

CHOOSING THE OPTION THAT'S RIGHT FOR YOU

Once you make your choice—lumpectomy, mastectomy, reconstruction or not—don't look back. You can always get a mastectomy later if you don't feel comfortable living with your lumpectomy. You can always get reconstruction later, too, or remove it if you prefer to go natural. Don't think that the decisions you made in those early days of diagnosis are set in stone. Anything, with the exception of mastectomy, can be changed.

Talk to your doctor about the options that are available to you. Some women opt for a bilateral mastectomy no matter how advanced their cancer is because they want their breasts *gone*. They don't want to take the risk of cancer showing up in their contralateral breast a few years down the road. They don't ever want to deal with any of this again. Other women don't have a choice. Their cancer is such that they have no alternative *but* a mastectomy. If this is true for you, your decision is already made. You have to do what is necessary to rid yourself of this disease, and getting yourself as far away from those cancer cells is, above all, the most important thing to focus on when you are panicking or mourning the loss of your breasts.

Regardless of which option you choose, you should mourn your loss. You don't look the same. You don't feel the same. And when you are in the midst of chemo, it is hard to see anything in a positive light. After treatment and your surgeries, though, you have to learn to accept the changes. But if there's something you truly don't like, do whatever is necessary to get the look you want.

LUMPECTOMY

Lumpectomy is the easier surgery . . . or so we are told. In reality, there is no such thing as an easy surgery when it comes to someone cutting into your breasts. A simple, uncomplicated lumpectomy can leave you with a small scar, but you remain somewhat intact. A deeper lumpectomy can leave a divot or a larger scar.

The survival rates for lumpectomies are only equal to those of mastectomies if the lumpectomy is followed by radiation. And radiation can cause changes in your breast. Your radiated breast will look different from your non-radiated breast, because radiation causes skin changes. One of the changes is the color. You will be tan on one side and pale on the other—think of a black and white cookie. The best way to counteract this look is to use a self tanner on paleface. Then you'll at least have a matched set. The radiated breast will also be firmer and tighter. There is really nothing you can do about that, though, unless you get the other one lifted.

If you have been in Cancerland for awhile, you have probably accumulated scars from previous biopsies. This can complicate lumpectomies and sometimes turn them into quadrectomies, instead. A quadrectomy is exactly what it sounds like—a quadrant of your breast is removed. Like a big piece of pie, a slice is taken from your breast. Additionally, if you have a deep or large tumor, or your margins are hard to clear, you may be left with a divot. While you can't really do anything about the scars from previous biopsies, you can have reconstructive surgery to fill in any quadrants that may need to be removed, and you can also get divots filled. Do not be shy about asking for any this if you are not pleased with the way your breasts look post-surgery.

MASTECTOMY

Mastectomies scare the hell out of everyone. How can they not? We agonize for years during adolescence about wanting our breasts to grow. At some point we might have even chanted, "We must, we must, we must increase our bust . . ." while making chicken dance movements with our arms. And now one of them is going to be taken away? After all the money we have spent on Wonderbras can this really be happening?

This feeling passes, of course, because you eventually realize that your once beloved breast is harboring terrorist cancer cells seeking to destroy you. Once you acknowledge that, you can't wait to get your breast off. As a matter of fact, you may want to take the other one off, too. When your basic survival instinct kicks in, it is amazing what you are capable of doing.

Mastectomies are constantly improving, and there are now skin-sparing mastectomies in which, as the name implies, doctors are able to preserve the skin. First, the breast tissue is removed from the underside of the skin, like taking the "meat" out of an avocado. The surgeon then removes the breast tissue that is to the side of your breast, along your rib cage. In addition to the skin, the chest muscle is now spared, as well. In the past, radical mastectomies used to remove most, if not all of the muscle, leaving women with a great deal of weakness and disfigurement. Thankfully, medicine has improved since then.

A mastectomy scar is usually horizontal and is proportionate to the size of the breast that was removed—the smaller your breast, the smaller your scar. No matter what size your scar is, take care of it. Don't expose it to the sun, because if you do, it won't fade; it will actually become more noticeable. Do, however, massage it every night with lotion or vitamin E oil. This can break it down, which will make it thinner. If you have raised scars or keloids, there are silicone scar patches you can get from either your doctor or specialty pharmacies. The patches will flatten and smooth your scar, but they won't make it disappear. Put in the work now, and you will be happier with your appearance later.

BILATERAL MASTECTOMY

Bilateral mastectomies are done for two reasons. The first is if there is cancer in both breasts that needs to be removed. The second is if the patient is removing the cancer-free breast for cosmetic and/or prophylactic reasons. Many women who carry the breast cancer gene opt for bilateral prophylactic mastectomies to prevent breast cancer from ever happening to them.

If you get both of your breasts removed and choose to reconstruct, you will have a better end result because you will have a matching set. This may seem like a lot to take in when making your surgical choices, but down the road when you are faced with a mix-matched pair you may wish you had done them both at the same time.

When making your decision, remember that even though your breasts may be taken away, the cancer that was inside of them will be taken away, as well. A great deal of comfort can come from knowing that your breasts, which were once harboring mutant DNA that was aimed at taking over your body, are now in a lab somewhere, far away from you. Now, the healing can begin.

CHOOSING NOT TO RECONSTRUCT

Your decisions aren't over after you've chosen your surgery. You still need to decide what you're going to do after the surgery is over. Will you remain natural? Will you reconstruct? What type of reconstruction will you choose? This is a big decision, so it's important to be well-informed about all of the available options. There is much to discuss, beginning with what life will be like if you choose not to reconstruct.

Prostheses

If you get a mastectomy and do nothing afterward, you will be left with one natural breast and one flat side where your breast used to be. Oftentimes, your doctor will leave you some extra skin. This offers you the opportunity for reconstruction should you choose it down the road, and it will also help give you the appearance of some cleavage with the proper prosthesis in place.

Finding a perfect fit for your prosthesis is important. You will be tender post-surgery, so you should only wear a soft filler made for post-surgical use. After your skin has healed, you can then get fitted for the right size, shape, and weight. This "evens" you out and helps to prevent a strain on your shoulders and neck, because you won't have the weight of only one breast pulling you out of alignment.

There are special prostheses for swimming. Make sure, though, that you have yours securely fastened to your suit because "swimmies" have been known to break free and cause some uncomfortable situations. No one wants their prosthetic to be unknowingly bobbing in the pool a few feet away from them while they're happily conversing with their boss's wife! To avoid circumstances such as this one, some women even attach a tether to their swimmie—kind of like surfers do with their boards—so they can reel it in on the off chance it makes a break for it.

Bras

Just because you have a prosthesis doesn't meant that you have start wearing industrial strength bras that look like they were designed for the Soviet Female Wrestling Team. There are beautiful mastectomy bras, and you can also buy silky, lacey bras that you can have a cup sewn into for your prosthesis. The better quality your mastectomy boutique, the more options you have. Don't skimp here. A good bra that makes you feel like *you* can make a tremendous difference emotionally. And by the way, please note that prostheses are covered under insurance. So get a good bra, or five. You are worth it. Make sure you buy a few pairs of matching panties to go with each bra you buy, too! More on that later . . .

Tiny Dancer Phenomenon

There is a special phenomenon that happens to a woman who has both breasts removed and no reconstruction. Rather than feeling less feminine, which is what one might assume, she feels *more* feminine. Think of Degas' paintings of the ballerinas. They have little to no breasts and are elegant, graceful, and as feminine a figure as you can find.

Also, take a look at the art from the 1920s by artists such as Erte and Mucha. They do not emphasize breasts. Instead, the inherent and unmistaken beauty of the entire feminine figure is celebrated. The women depicted often have big eyes, long graceful arms, and beautiful clothing. Back then, the bosom was not the blistering beacon it is in today's media. The media of today focuses on "ideal" things that everyone is supposed to fall in lockstep to meet, regardless of whether they are healthy or safe. Keep in mind that the same media that tells us big breasts are feminine, is also encouraging women to have their genitals reconstructed to look more "appealing." How we got to this point is beyond reason. J. Algernon Hawthorne, in the classic 1968 movie, *It's a Mad, Mad, Mad, Mad World*, summed it up beautifully:

> This infantile preoccupation with bosoms! In all my time in this Godforsaken country, the one thing that has appalled me most of all is this preposterous preoccupation with bosoms. Don't you realize they have become the dominant theme in American culture: in literature, advertising and all fields of entertainment and

everything. I'll wager you anything you like that if American women stopped wearing brassieres, your whole national economy would collapse overnight.

How true!

Benefit of Picking Your Size

One of the benefits of not reconstructing and going without breasts is the opportunity to start from scratch. If you had a bilateral mastectomy, you can choose any size you want to be in a breast form. For instance, if you always wanted to be a C cup, you can get C cup-sized breast forms. If, on the other hand, you were always large-chested, exercise that you couldn't do before is now an option for you. Running and tennis are a lot more fun when you don't have to wear two bras because your breasts are so large. Many women like having the choice of going with or without their breast forms, depending on their mood or activity.

CHOOSING TO RECONSTRUCT

Your breast surgeon takes away. He takes away your breasts, but he also takes away the cancer. His job is to make certain that there are no cancer cells lurking, so he removes as much breast tissue as possible. Even though he is in the Removal Department, he is also in the Giving Department. Because of his work, your life very well may be saved, which is evidenced by the fact that 70 percent of all breast cancers are cured by surgery alone. If that statistic doesn't make you pick the best breast specialist you can find, what will?

Your plastic surgeon falls at the other end of the spectrum. He is kind of like Santa Claus. You go to sleep on his table and wake up to find beautiful presents under the bandages he has wrapped you in. He gives you back what had to be taken away to save your life.

Before that can happen, though, you have a lot of choices to make. Do you get implants or do you use fat from another part of your body? And where in your body do you want that fat to come from? How you choose depends on many factors: the state of your health, how much fat you have at a donor site, how much surgery you want to endure, and what you want your end result to look like. It's also important to understand that no reconstruction is immediate. When you decide to reconstruct, you become a work in progress —an *artwork* in progress. It's a process and there is fine tuning that must be done along the way. Breaking down the types of reconstruction should help you understand what, exactly, the process entails.

Implants

An implant is a two-step procedure. First, a tissue expander is inserted, and then it is followed by an implant at a later date. An implant requires a tissue expander to create a pocket behind the pectoral muscle for the implant to be placed. The expander is an empty "balloon" that has a metal port connected to it. After your initial healing, you visit your doctor's office for "fills." The doctor accesses the metal port by locating it with a magnet. Then, the expander is filled with saline solution in small increments, which stretches the skin. There is some discomfort in this procedure, as there will be a feeling of tightness in the chest area. But over-the-counter pain relievers will usually alleviate the pain.

When the plastic surgeon is satisfied with the amount of room now available under the skin and muscle, you go in for your "exchange" surgery. This means exchanging the temporary expander with your permanent implant. You will have to decide between saline implants and silicone implants. Saline implants have the feeling of a water balloon, whereas silicone implants have a more natural feeling. The newer, cohesive, gel implants are made of a silicone that is in a gel form. This not only offers a better cosmetic appearance, but there is no risk of silicone leakage because even if you cut the implant in half, the gel stays stationary and does not ooze or travel. Of all the reconstruction options, expander to implant is the easiest, the least painful, and requires the least amount of recovery time.

Do you think you can't get implants because of prior radiation? If so, you need to think again. There is a new product called AlloDerm, which is made from donor tissue that has been stripped of all of its

DNA. When implanted under a woman's breast pocket, it heals as part of her own tissue, taking on her DNA. It creates a type of support similar to a hammock that supports the implant. It also strengthens the skin, making it possible for even previously radiated skin able to support an implant. Not all doctors are up to date on its uses, but as its success stories grow, more reconstructive surgeons are learning how to use AlloDerm, and as a result, more women will have this option in breast reconstruction. So, if you are thinking of getting reconstruction but were told that because you had radiation, implants are not possible, you now know that to be false. You just have to find the right doctor.

Implants are a quick fix. They offer a short recovery time, require less time in the operating room than other reconstructive options, and pleasantly result in round, perky breasts. However, some women do not like the look or feel of implants. They can be firm to the touch and they are located under the pectoral muscles. Because of this location, when you flex your muscles you get what is known as "animation" in your breasts. Essentially, your pecs push your implants down and make them look like they are moving or contracting.

Another undesirable outcome with implants is rippling and puckering, which is caused by the thin layer of skin laying over the implants. If you are a slim person, you will see the puckering through your skin. There are, however, new implants in clinical trial right now that are firmer and wider at the bottom than they are at the top, and thus, they do not cause rippling. Be sure to ask your doctor about this new option.

The final drawback of implant reconstruction is the possibility of capsular contracture. Your body may create scar tissue around the foreign objects—the implants—which will tighten the capsules that hold them. This pushes the implants higher and causes pain. The only way to correct this complication is by removing the scar tissue and replacing the implants.

Flap Procedures, With and Without Muscle

If you do not want to use implants, you still have many beautiful options. They are more surgically involved, but they offer stunning results. By using tissue from another part of your body in what is known as a flap procedure, you can have soft, warm, natural-feeling breasts that look as close to the real thing as you can get. This is a durable reconstruction, meaning that your new breasts will gain and lose weight when you do and they will last a lifetime. All of this comes at a price, though. Using your own tissue will make for a longer surgery, a longer recovery, and a scar on another part of your body.

Flap procedures, also known as autogulous reconstruction, are performed by plastic surgeons who are experienced in micro-surgery. Tissue for the flap can be taken from the back, the abdomen, the buttocks, or the inner thigh. Some procedures take muscle and fat along with the skin, but others are "free flaps" and leave the muscle in place. No matter where the flap is taken from, you should expect to be in the operating room for many hours, to stay in the hospital for at least four days, and to have a long recovery that is eventually followed up with more surgery to tweak the final results.

During the initial surgery, the flap of skin, fat, and muscle, if necessary, is removed from the donor site with the blood vessels intact. That site is then closed and the surgeons begin to work on the breast creation. Next, the chest is prepared. Sometimes a section of rib must be removed to access the blood vessels of the chest. The flap is then put into place with the micro-surgery connecting the exposed blood vessels. Once completed, the surgeon forms the shape of the breast and closes the area. The tissue that used to be part of your back, belly, buttocks, or thigh, is now two round, soft, breasts with their own blood supply. They feel natural and will look natural when all the healing is complete.

While flap procedures may take longer, cause more pain, and have a longer recovery time, the end result is breasts that feel and look like your old breasts. Also, if the donor site was your belly, you have gotten a tummy tuck; if it was your butt, it is now smaller; and if it was your thigh, you have an instant thigh lift. Not a bad trade off!

Now that you know the basics about flap procedures in general, let's talk a little more specifically about all of the different kinds.

Latissimus Dorsi Flap

A latissimus dorsi flap, or LD flap, takes the latissimus dorsi muscle from the back and brings it around to the chest. The blood vessels are attached and you are left with a new breast that has its own blood supply. Many times, an implant is added to increase the cup size. But unlike implants alone that have just have a thin layer of skin over them, the LD flap adds tissue, making the skin thicker and more viable for better nipple creation.

The donor site is just under the shoulder blade and the scar is anywhere from six to fourteen inches long. You will require two or three follow-up surgeries to do the fine tuning on the beautiful end result. These include exchanging the tissue expander for an implant, adding nipples and areolas, and correcting anything that is not symmetrical.

If you are athletic, particularly if you are a swimmer or tennis player, this surgery will affect your ability to enjoy activities the way you did before. This is the trade-off for the LD flap; you gain a breast, but you lose a muscle that helped you exercise, making you weaker and unable to attain the same level of endurance or strength that you had before the surgery.

There is also a rare complication that can sometimes accompany an LD flap, where the nerves of the muscle start to regenerate. When this happens, every time you move your arms, the muscle that is now your breast contracts and flattens your chest. If this occurs, more surgery is required to sever the nerves and make the muscle immobile. With this added surgery, there is a risk of losing the blood supply, which would result in the loss of your entire reconstructed breast.

You must discuss this possible complication with your doctor before you opt to have an LD flap procedure. Be sure to explain your current level of activity, and tell him you do not want to lose the ability to do the things you enjoy, like swimming or tennis.

Transverse Rectus Abdominis Myocutaeous Flap

The TRAM flap was once the most popular reconstructive surgery involving the use of a woman's own tissue. The downside, however, is that it causes a loss of abdominal muscle. TRAM flaps slide the abdominal muscle, fat, and a main blood vessel up your torso, over your rib cage, and into the place of your breast on your chest wall.

You have two surgical sites when you are through, and both need time to heal. Your abdomen will take extra time to heal due to the loss of muscle. The scar goes across your abdomen from hip to hip, and you will require further surgeries to correct any imperfections or asymmetry, as well as to add the nipples and areolas. This is a more involved surgery than the implant or LD flap, and it requires a long period of recuperation. The plus side is a warm, realistic-looking breast with the added benefit of a tummy tuck.

TRAM flaps create beautiful breasts. However, many patients do not want to lose their entire abdominal muscle, because that can cause weaknesses, such as hernias and lower back problems that affect quality of life. Doctors have now perfected ways of using small amounts of muscle instead of the entire rectus abdominis, which has made the surgery far better and much more appealing to women. However, because of the complications that can arise from moving and removing muscle, the procedure of choice now is a free flap, where a flap is taken from either the abdomen or the buttocks.

Deep Inferior Epigastric Perforator Flap

You want only a board certified reconstructive surgeon who is experienced in micro-vascular surgery to perform this type of flap. In this procedure, fat and micro-vascular tissue are removed from the abdomen, leaving the rectus abdominis muscle in place. Rather than removing the abdominal muscle, the surgeon carefully pulls out the perforator vessels that will carry the blood supply to the flap once it is attached to the chest. The blood vessels are then reconnected and the fat is shaped into a soft, pliable, extremely real-istic-looking breast.

Because of the intricacy of this operation, it takes longer than the implant, LD flap, and TRAM flap. However, you have an easier healing process with this procedure than you do with the TRAM flap procedure because the muscle is spared. You also get a large portion of fat removed from your abdomen, which gives you the added benefit of a tummy tuck. If you don't need a tummy tuck or if you don't have enough fat to spare around the middle, your buttocks can be used.

Gluteal Artery Perforator Flap

A gluteal flap, or GAP flap, procedure is a free flap procedure where the excess fat from your buttocks is used to make the breast. The cut is made just below the bikini line on the butt and the fat is removed along with the perforator blood vessels of the gluteal muscle. This flap is then brought to your chest wall and the vessels are reattached, providing a soft, natural-shaped breast.

There are two GAP flap options. An I-GAP, or inferior gluteal artery perforator flap, takes tissue from the bottom of your buttocks. The scar will be "hidden" in the crease where your leg meets your butt cheek. An S-GAP, or superior gluteal artery perforator flap, takes tissue from the upper portion of your buttocks, almost like a shark bite. Your surgeon will fill in any defects or divots this procedure causes at a later date.

You begin the surgery positioned on your stomach so the surgeon can remove the tissue from the buttocks. You are then turned over so the reconstruction of the breast can begin. It is a long procedure, and the best way to have it done is to have two doctors performing it at the same time. This reduces the length of time you are under anesthesia, as well as decreases the risk of your flap losing viability while they are closing the buttock incision.

After you have healed, a revision is done, where the surgeon goes back to the butt and lifts it, creating a new and better looking derriere. If you have always dreamed of getting a better butt and no amount of exercise has helped—and you just happen to need two, new, life-like breasts made from your own tissue—this may be the option for you.

Transverse Upper Gracilis Flap

The TUG flap takes the fat of the inner thigh along with the gracilis muscle to form a breast. Like the other flap procedures, it requires a delicate, micro-surgical technique, as well as subsequent surgeries to fine tune and add the nipples and areolas. The advantage of the TUG procedure over the GAP procedure is that you do not have to be turned over during surgery. This makes life easier for the surgeons and helps to keep the flap viable since it is exposed for a shorter amount of time.

The gracilis muscle is used in many reconstructive procedures, and the loss of this muscle is not a factor in quality of life or mobility after the surgery. The muscle and tissue are brought up to the breast area and the blood vessels are connected. Because of the elongated shape of the gracilis muscle, the surgeon can create a breast with more projection than the other flap procedures allow.

The scar on the thigh either runs along the crease of the upper leg or down the inner thigh, depending on the volume of tissue available. If you have more fat lower on your leg, then the surgeon will use a lateral incision, meaning it will be vertical instead of horizontal. Regardless, the end result is a thigh lift.

Even though this procedure is lesser known than some of the others, it is gaining popularity. The gracilis muscle creates a beautiful breast and the surgery is easier than some of the others. Additionally, many women who do not have enough abdominal fat or who have had previous abdominal surgery are now choosing this great new option.

Realistic Expectations with Your Reconstruction

No matter what kind of procedure you choose, you will initially be swollen, in pain, and feel like aliens have landed on your chest. It will feel as raw and harsh as you imagined it would. After all, each of the procedures involve a major surgery on a part of your body that is very intimately connected to your femininity. There will be scars, bandages, and drains, and it won't be pretty.

Luckily, things get better! This reconstructive process also has a middle and an end. The middle part is when the swelling begins to go down. The raised red scars also smooth out and get lighter in color. And, when you look down, you see cleavage. You don't know *whose* cleavage, but it is there! This brings us to the disconnect that is often felt by reconstructed women. We don't feel like our new breasts are a part of us yet. They are like rental cars. We know how to drive them, they operate the same way as our own cars, but they don't look the same, smell the same, or feel the same. And what's more, we feel like everyone who looks at us *knows* we are "renting" them.

The middle part of the reconstructive process is also the time of revisions and tweaking. You may have your tissue expanders exchanged for the final implants, or you may have the final nips and tucks done to complete your flap construction. Things start to look better. You get used to being in your new skin, literally. You have gotten the hang of what tops look good and you know what kind of bras to wear—or, you discover that you never have to wear one again. You also find yourself looking in the mirror and admiring what you see!

The end of the process makes all the difference in the world. Don't go through all of this work and then not finish the job. Put the icing on the cake! Get your nipples and areolas done. Then, when they heal get them tattooed to match the color that your old ones were. When this procedure is done and you see your new breasts, complete with nipples, there is a sense of coming home. You feel like *you* again. You see yourself as real again. You may never accept the new breasts as yours completely, but this finishing touch can do more for you psychologically than anything else. When you get nipples and areolas, your scars seem to disappear, which is definite bonus. Also, when you look down at your chest and see nipples after seeing Barbie-like smooth bumps for so long, you get a jolt of recognition—a feeling of, "Oh my! I remember those!" And that feeling alone is worth the surgery.

PERSONAL STORY: JESSICA CLEANS UP

Jessica had cancer in both of her breasts. She had always loved her breasts and felt they were one of her best features, so when the doctors told her she had no alternative but a bilateral mastectomy, she felt as if the very essence of her being was going to be taken away. But then she saw her MRI report. She saw that she had both ductal and lobular tumors. She saw that the breasts she adored might literally kill her, and suddenly she couldn't wait to have the surgery.

Before the big day, Jessica had to go to the reconstructive surgeon's office and get marked for her tissue expanders. Then, it was off to the hospital. As she undressed and put on her hospital gown, she looked down at her beautiful breasts for the last time.

Eight hours later she woke up from surgery. When she was fully conscious, the first thing she did was look at her chest. She wasn't flat. She saw two mounds under the hospital gown. If she didn't know any better, she would have thought they left her breasts in place. When she was finally allowed out of bed, she slowly made it to the bathroom. She opened the gown and saw a surgical bra and a lot of gauze padding. She also saw cleavage.

Somewhat to her surprise, Jessica's heart was not heavy. She felt clean—clean for the first time since this whole nightmare started. The cancer was now off of her and she had new breasts somewhere under there. It was then that she knew she would be able to handle anything anyone threw at her.

PART TWO

---

*Y*our Sexual
Reclamation

You were a beautiful, sexy woman before breast cancer entered your life. But then your doctor told you that you had a life-threatening disease and everything changed. You were confused because although you had a lump in your breast, you didn't feel sick. The diagnosis seemed to come out of nowhere. You were then hit with the news that you would lose all or part of that breast, and that you would have to start chemotherapy, which meant you were going to lose your hair, too. You quickly discovered that you were also going to have to feel really sick in order to get better. What happened? You were feeling fine the previous week, but now? Not so much.

Throughout your treatments you did everything the doctors told you to do. You flew through surgeries and could strip a drain like no one's business. You rocked your bald head and either got a bodacious wig or became the queen of hats and scarves—or you said the hell with it and showed the world what a beautiful bald woman looks like. After the chemo rid your body of cancer, the radiation clean-up crew finished the job and your plastic surgeon, if you went that route, started to perform magic on you by rebuilding your body.

Now that you are post-treatment, you're most likely beginning to see your hair grow back. But you're probably also noticing that you've put on weight. Those not-so-funny jokes about what a great "diet" cancer is turned out to be a lie. You look in the mirror and see lines where there used to be none. You may have been hurled into early menopause and you also notice that you haven't had the remotest interest in sex in quite some time. You look at your body— your newly, reconstructed body—and there is a disconnect. Your new "girls" may be perfect specimens of a reconstructive surgeon's art and talent, they may be perkier than an eighteen-year-old's, and they may look like something out of a Victoria's Secret Catalog, but they are not *yours*. Who is that in the mirror? And how can she ever feel desirable again when she cannot even reconcile her own sense of self?

To add insult to injury, your sexual organs don't seem to be working right either. You have vaginal dryness and discomfort, and if you've feebly attempted to make love it was most likely so painful that it resulted in tears, embarrassment, and guilt. What happened? Just last year you were hot and sexy! Just last year you loved making love! Just last year you finally decided that you didn't give a crap about your cellulite—the rest of you was good enough to overcome a few dimpled cheeks! What the hell happened?

If this sounds like you, if any of this strikes a nerve, it should bring you comfort; because, you see, you are not the only one feeling this way. *All* women who have fought the battle you just fought feel like this in some form or another. Don't let cancer rob you of happiness, just keep moving forward. You did not fight for your life to live with self-loathing and only memories of a passionate sex life.

The time to reclaim *you* is now. The woman you were before cancer is still inside of you and this second part of the book is going to teach you how to get her out. Your body escaped Cancerland, so now it's time to let your mojo-loving, drop-dead-gorgeous goddess get the hell out of there, too.

You *can* get your desire back.
You *can* get your mojo back.
You *can* get your body working like it used to.
You *can* feel great about how you look again.
You *can* live the life you fought so hard to keep.

Girl, get off the Cancerland bus. Slip into something slinky. You are going to love *you* again. And here is how you are going to do it.

6

*R*eclaiming Your Sexuality

Okay, so you have physical, emotional, and mental obstacles to overcome. Now that you are faced with newly discovered sexual problems, it all may seem too daunting to conquer. Remember: You defeated *cancer*. You can handle the aftermath. Yes, it takes time. But if you are determined, anything is possible. Now is the time to attack what is happening to the sexual aspects of your body and your mind. We begin with how to overcome what is physically affecting your sexuality.

EARLY MENOPAUSE

If you get breast cancer before you are in menopause, chances are the chemo will kick you into it, the Tamoxifen will make you feel like you are in it, or your doctor will advise you that you need a prophylactic oophrectomy—the removal of your ovaries—to surgically put you in it. Studies have shown that in estrogen-receptor positive women, removing all sources of estrogen is a beneficial idea. Ovaries, this means you. Also, if you are a high-risk patient, meaning you have a strong family history of both breast and ovarian cancer, or you carry the BRCA gene, your ovaries are going to be facing deportation. Keep in mind that you have a higher risk of ovarian cancer because of your breast cancer, as well. All this will mean a farewell to the ovaries and a baptism by hot flash into the world of sudden menopause.

When your ovaries are shut down or removed, you will experience hot flashes, moodiness, and even some sexual side effects. These include a decreased libido, vaginal dryness, and vaginal atrophy, which can make intercourse painful, if not impossible. Compound that with cancer treatments and multiple surgeries, and romance may be the last thing on your mind. As you may have already discovered, there is quite a lot to overcome here.

Lucikly, there are things that can help you after you go through chemo-pause or ovary removal that throws you into an early menopause. Your quality of life is important, so you need to know about all of them—especially if you're an estrogen-dependent breast cancer patient. If you are, you cannot pop a Prempro or other hormone replacement drug, because they encourage the growth of breast cancer. So, how do you feel better when there are so many things that are not permitted? When a door closes a window opens. The following information breaks down what is safe, what works, and what you can do, naturally, to help improve your mood, desire, hot flashes, and life.

THE IMPORTANCE OF YOUR DIET

You don't always have to reach for a pill to get the nutrients you need—although they can sometimes be beneficial. You can, instead, make small dietary changes that will have a significant impact. For instance, you can increase your intake of Omega-3 fatty acids by eating deep water fish. The oil actually improves your skin texture and helps counteract vaginal dryness. In addition, switching to a plant-based diet rich in whole foods and whole grains will provide a gateway to health by naturally supplying your body with beta-carotene, calcium, the B vitamins, and vitamins C and E. Conversely, there are certain things you should avoid, including soy and black cohosh. Take the time to learn about these naturally-occurring products and your body will thank you.

Flaxseed

Flaxseed is an excellent addition to your diet. Whole, cold-milled, ground flaxseed, put into your food, can add lignans and Omega-3 fatty acids to your diet. It may also help prevent recurrence of triple-negative breast cancer—the type of breast cancer that is not fueled by estrogen or progesterone. Ground flaxseeds are superior to flaxseed oil, and have been studied in hormone-sensitive breast cancer, as well. Some studies show that ground flaxseeds can decrease tumor size and reduce breast cancer recurrence. Sprinkle a few tablespoons in your morning cereal or in your yogurt. Go easy at first, because it can make your GI tract a little more active than normal. It is best to ease into the regimen.

Vitamin E

Vitamin E not only helps with hot flashes, but it also helps your skin stay young. Additionally, it can help your libido and aid in keeping delicate vaginal tissues supple. Taking vitamin E with hot water and lemon, or cool lemonade made from real lemons—not a mix—has been shown to reduce hot flashes. You can also combine vitamin E with 1,000 milligrams of vitamin C for the same effect. For vitamin E dosing, never take more than 200 IUs in a day. And even then, it is best to break up the dose: 50 to 100 IUs in the morning, and 50 to 100 IUs in the evening. Another great use for vitamin E is as a lubricant for your vaginal tissues. Some women insert a daily capsule to combat dryness and atrophy, while others apply the oil topically, directly to their skin. If you have heart disease or you are on blood thinners, check with your doctor before using any vitamin E, because it may not be safe for you.

Beta Carotene

Beta carotene is the same thing as vitamin A. It helps with vaginal dryness and can also increase your skin's elasticity if you are showing signs of premature aging. The American Heart Association and the American Cancer Society warn that the safest way to get beta carotene is through diet, rather than through supplementation. Five servings of fruits and vegetables daily, plus a diet high in whole grains, provides six to eight milligrams of beta-carotene. There are no recommended doses for vitamin A/beta carotene because of this. But if you must take a supplement, the safest dosage is the lowest: 15 milligrams a day, by mouth, for adults.

The B Vitamins

B vitamins are very popular and can help with vaginal dryness, fatigue, stress, and mood swings. However, there can be too much of a good thing. For instance, high doses of B_6 can cause nerve pain, whereas lower, correct doses can combat neuropathy—the nerve pain brought on by chemotherapy. Thus, in this instance, more does not equal better. Stick to a B-Complex 50 combination, which combines all the B vitamins you need in a controlled dose of no more than 50 milligrams. If you are eating a good diet of whole foods—meaning whole grains, unprocessed, plant-based foods, eggs, and beans—you are getting a natural source of B vitamins, which is always the best way. More good news: recent studies have shown that the combination of vitamin B_{12} and folate can reduce breast cancer risk.

Calcium

Calcium is vital to your future bone health, and it may even help fight cancer recurrence. Take 1,200 milligrams each day. Add magnesium to that, or take a calcium with magnesium added to its formulation, and it will help fight fatigue and keep you regular—if you find that calcium supplements without magnesium cause constipation.

Evening Primrose Oil

Evening primrose oil is a good source of gamma linoleic acid (GLA), and it has been used by many women to help vaginal dryness. However, its side effects include increased bleeding, so if you are on seizure medication or anticoagulants, it should not be used. Evening primrose oil can also cause GI upset, headache, and a host of other complaints, so be careful with it. It is best used topically on vaginal tissues, rather than taken internally. See page 86 for more information on vaginal moisturizers and lubricants.

Melatonin

Melatonin not only helps you sleep, but it may also help fight cancer recurrence. If you are having trouble with insomnia due to lack of estrogen, taking melatonin before bed may help. Speak with your doctor about the proper dose for you.

Omega-3 Fatty Acids

Foods that are high in Omega-3 fatty acids can help boost your libido, help your skin, and even combat hot flashes. Wild salmon is the best source of Omega-3s, but olive oil, nuts, and avocados will all help keep your skin and vaginal tissues supple, as well. And yes, chocolate has been proven to be an all-around mood and libido booster, and a powerful anti-oxidant. Yeah baby!

Soy

Soy is rich in phytoestrogens, which means it is a plant estrogen. Many women are told by their doctors *not* to add soy to their diets if they have hormone-sensitive breast cancer. This is because it can act like an estrogen and possibly affect the efficacy of hormone-blocking drugs taken to prevent breast cancer recurrence. A high intake of soy can also affect your thyroid, which is not good if you are on a thyroid medication. There once was a study that said soy reduced breast cancer, but that study was overturned and replaced by one that said it could *promote* breast cancer. After all you have been through, do you really want to play Russian Roulette with a supplement that the "experts" think may make you suffer a breast cancer recurrence? There are other, less-risky, natural ways to supplement your diet and reduce the symptoms of hot flashes, mood swings, low libido, and vaginal dryness. Speak with your doctor and ask if you should opt for those instead.

Black Cohosh

In a word, no. Avoid black cohosh. Yes, there are studies after studies about how it helps everything from hot flashes to libido. However, similar to soy, you should stay away from it if you have estrogen-sensitive breast cancer. It has been found to be a possible cause of the growth of breast cancer tumors. Ask your oncologist.

MEDICATIONS THAT CAN AFFECT YOUR LIBIDO

With all this natural goodness, you may still find that nothing works. Why? Because you are on medications that counteract everything else you are doing to improve your life. These include medications your doctor has prescribed to help prevent a breast cancer recurrence, to improve your mood, or to ease your anxiety. While your doctor is trying to help you and your quality of life, the sexual side of your life often pays the price in adverse side effects. Once you know what can kill your libido, you can talk to your doctor about making some changes.

Selective Serotonin Re-Uptake Inhibitors (SSRIs)

This is the largest group of antidepressants that are prescribed. They work directly on nerve endings, and many doctors give them to breast cancer survivors to help the depression that may follow their long, arduous therapy. Some of these drugs have also been known to help with the lingering after-effects of chemo and estrogen loss. Unfortunately, the most common side effect is loss of sexual libido. Since these types of antidepressants alter your serotonin level, and serotonin plays a big part of sexual function, it's no wonder they kill your libido. The good news is that not all antidepressants are SSRIs. Medications like Wellbutrin, for example, do not affect the libido, nor do they make you gain weight, as some SSRIs tend to do. So, be sure to talk to your doctor about your options and determine what is best for you.

Tranquilizers

Valium, Librium, and Xanax, which all work on the limbic area of the brain by sedating the sensory nerves and pleasure pathways, can cause sexual side effects such as loss of libido. They are also known to cause an inability to reach orgasm. Time your dosing around when you are planning on making love if you need to. In other words, don't take that Xanax during the few hours before intimacy, or you may not achieve a satisfying experience.

Pain Medications

Drugs that are taken to kill pain also kill sensation, make you drowsy, and reduce your libido and enjoyment of sex, for obvious reasons. Common opioids, such as Codeine, Percocette, and others, as well as newer drugs being prescribed for chemo-induced neuropathy, like Neurontin, are libido killers. Unfortunately, many cancer survivors are on pain killers for a long time—long after the pain has abated. The surgery has healed and the chemo side effects have lessened or disappeared, but they are still taking heavy-duty pain meds. Doctors suggest a weaning off of the narcotic medication slowly, and supplementing with over-the-counter medication, like Tylenol or Advil, instead. You may find that you feel better once the fog of opiates is gone from your body, and that your pain is more than manageable or non-existant.

Cold and Allergy Medicines

Over-the-counter medicines for colds, coughs, and allergies can zonk you out, as well as dry you out. You don't need that! The lesson is to be aware of side effects from all your medications, not just the ones that are prescribed. There are natural ways to clear a stopped up nose and help with allergies. The most effective is a saline rinse that you can buy in any pharmacy. It is spritzed into each nostril and can clear your stuffy nose. It can even ease sinus pain. Studies have also shown that over-the-counter cough medicines don't work any better than a cup of tea with honey and lemon, so try that first. It breaks up congestion, tastes good, and doesn't dry out every part of your body.

Non-Steroidal Anti-Inflammatory Drugs (NSAIDS)

Drugs like Advil and Alleve reduce lubrication and kill desire. You might want to try a Tylenol instead because it doesn't have those side effects. Just be cautious with how much alcohol you consume when taking it, because it has been known to cause liver problems when taken with excessive amounts.

Multiple Medical Problems (MMP)

If you have multiple medical problems—and who doesn't after a cancer diagnosis and treatment—then you qualify as MMP. This means that you are taking many different drugs for many different reasons, which can compound side effects in all aspects. Not only that, but the drug combo you are on can also kill your sexual desire, your arousal, and your ability to orgasm. If this is happening to you, sit down with your doctor and go over everything you are taking to figure out what is robbing you of your mojo. All of your conditions should be evaluated bi-annually. You may find that you no longer require the drugs you were prescribed two years ago. And the less you take, the better you will feel.

THE LIBIDO HORIZON

There is emerging research being done on women's lack of sexual desire and ways to overcome it. This is not just breast cancer survivors, either. Many women suffer from a shift in desire at one time or another in their lives. Sometimes it is related to menopause, but other times it is just an internal shift that is disheartening for them and frustrating for their partners. When breast cancer survivors come out of treatment, they are loaded with chemicals, as well as emotional and physical pain, and it takes awhile for them to feel sexual again. But what all women need to know is that they do not have to live without desire or sex permanently.

The simple, self-affirmation techniques we discuss on page 169 to help with our self esteem can also be used to recharge our libido batteries. Visualize yourself as a sexual being, not as someone who is *no longer* a sexual being. Touch your body. Allow yourself to enjoy the sensations of putting on a body cream or taking a long, hot bath. Invent a "Mojo Mantra" to repeat to yourself to help boost your inner goddess. For instance, " I love to touch and to be touched, and I want to make love," or, " I am beautiful, desirable, and sexy," or something similar that will help you return to a desirous frame of mind. Then, take little vacations in your mind. Look at that cute guy you work with while he's sitting at his desk and imagine running your tongue along his neck muscles. Why not? Men do this to women every day in their minds, and fantasy is a wonderful way to give a jump start to your libido.

There is also a medication that may soon be available, which will help increase women's libidos. Where men take Viagra because they mentally want to have sex but physically cannot, women are often just the opposite. Their bodies will comply, but they have no desire whatsoever. That is where a drug called flibanserin may come in. It was being tested as a new antidepressant. It didn't work for depression, but the women in the study found that it did increase their desire and enjoyment of sex. So, now it is back in trial—this time, for lack of desire in women. Right now flibanserin is still considered investigational, but if the respondents' claims of "significant improvement" continue, there may finally be a "Viagra" for women. And researchers may want to rethink it "not working" as an antidepressant after all!

BREAST SENSATION—NUMBNESS AND PAIN

After your surgeries, you felt pain. Then, slowly, you healed. The swelling and pain subsided, and were replaced with *nothing*. Literally. Your once sensitive-to-the-touch breasts went numb.

It is normal to experience breast, chest, torso, and arm pain from radiation for some time after treatment. Your skin eventually heals, but then you may begin experiencing a sharp pain in your sternum. This is also very common, and is known as costochondritis. (You know you have this if you press on your chest, right between your breasts, and you feel pain that then disappears when you stop pressing.) It, too, is nothing to panic about and will eventually go away. If you notice swelling of your upper body or arm, though, see your doctor immediately because you may be developing a condition known as lymphedema (see page 10).

As you continue to heal and when the pain finally stops, you will be left with numbness. If you had a lumpectomy, the numbness is not so bad. But if you had a mastectomy with or without reconstruction, the sensation you once had is gone. Most women who get skin-sparing mastectomies are surprised that the sparing did not include the nerves. Even nipple-sparing mastectomies cause a loss of sensation. Logically, it makes sense because your surgeon had to remove a lot of tissue to rid your body of cancer. But, it is still very disorienting. We get used to our breasts being major players in the pleasure zones of our lives.

This numbness will not only affect your sex life, but it will impact your daily life, as well. You will have to learn to keep an eye on your chest if you are wearing something revealing. Because your breasts have lost sensation, your top can shift and you won't feel it—meaning you may accidentally reveal a lot more than you planned on and not know it. Many women have had no idea they were flashing kids at the pool until they looked down and saw their bikini tops had shifted without them feeling it.

HOW TO OVERCOME THE LOSS
OF BREAST SENSATION

It is hard to lose an erogenous zone like the breasts. But have you really lost it? Remember, your mind is mighty. It can compensate for just about anything. Even so, when you are with a man and he reaches for one of your breasts, chances are, you won't feel it. You can watch his hand cup it, but the shock waves you normally felt before you had cancer won't happen. He may be perplexed, as well, if he knows you can't feel what he is doing. After all, it has been one of the first moves in his repertoire for a long time and is part of of his pleasure zone, too. Now what is he supposed to do?

Your surgeon took away a good portion of skin and nerve endings, but not all. In fact, when you were sewn back up, a lot of your skin was simply lifted higher. Therefore, if you explore, you may find some incredible sensitivity around your collarbone and your neck. And asking your man to kiss your nerve-packed neck instead of your numb nipples is a win-win situation. He still has something erotic to do, and you will feel the shock waves again.

In short, the sensation that you used to feel and love in your breasts may be gone, but you can teach your partner how to find your new pleasure zones. That being said, you first have to find them yourself so you can then show him how and where to turn you on.

Exercise in Touch for You

Lie back, and with the eraser of a pencil, gently touch the skin under your collarbone. Slowly move the pencil around that entire area until you begin to feel a familiar sensation—one that is reminiscent of your old erogenous zone. Gently circle the eraser down to the top of your breasts. Move it slowly and enjoy the strokes. It is pleasurable and stimulating. Why? Because, as previously mentioned, your breast skin has been stretched and moved around a bit. And while you may be completely numb where your nipples and areolas are, you still have plenty of sensation around your breast, chest, collarbone, and neck.

Exercise in Touch for Both of You

How do you teach this to your lover? Let's face it, he is not going to want to listen to a long, technical explanation. Instead, show him. Men like to learn through show and tell. Have him sit in his underwear, and with the pencil eraser, make the exact same movements that you found pleasurable on yourself, on his inner thigh, up where it meets his torso. Chances are, he will find this extremely arousing— especially because you are not touching any other area.

Now, tell him to do to you what you just did to him. But have him use his fingers or tongue instead of the pencil eraser on the areas around your breasts where you found the nerve endings. This will take you to the high places you used to go when your original breasts were stimulated. The "Numb Factor" has now been conquered by a simple change in geography. Once you have shown your man what you like, he will go there. He may forget in the throes of passion and his wandering hand may naturally land on your breast, so pay attention. If it happens, take the time to once again show him where you do have sensation. Show and tell. Show and tell.

VAGINAL DRYNESS AND ATROPHY

In addition to the loss of breast sensation, other common side effects of cancer treatment are vaginal dryness and atrophy, which can make sex painful, if not impossible. Wasn't cancer bad enough? We have to get used to this, too? No! No, you have not been sentenced to a life without sex. Dryness and atrophy do not have to rule your future.

Let's cut to the chase: It is all reversible! Just because you may have less lubrication does not mean that your genital area has shut down completely. Your body still responds to stimulation and can still reach orgasm. All you need to do is make up for what is missing and continue on with your sex life—with the emphasis on *continue*. There are more menopausal women now than ever with healthy sex lives. The most important thing they did to achieve that was to not stop having sex. *That* is the secret.

If you don't have a partner, there are ways to compensate on your own. The worst thing you can do is nothing. This is a very important lesson, and unfortunately, our doctors do not discuss it with us. If they did, we would not go back to their offices months later complaining about a poor quality of life and the loss of our sex lives. If we only knew what we had to do to keep ourselves luscious, we would live much better lives! With that happy fact in mind, read on.

Vaginal Dryness

As estrogen levels decline, your skin's elasticity becomes weaker, thinner, and more fragile. This includes your facial skin, as well as the skin of your vagina. To help our faces, we use creams and lotions. To help our vaginas, we should do the same thing. Daily vaginal lubrication can stop dryness. There are many over-the-counter daily lubricants women can use. Some are for maintaining moisture, and others are for use during sex. They come in a variety of forms, as well—from the simple, like vitamin E oil, to the more complex over-the-counter pearls and long lasting lubricant gels.

Perhaps the most surprising of all the lubrication options has been in your grandmother's pantry for decades. Crisco vegetable shortening has secretly been used for daily lubrication by breast cancer survivors for years. Men have their little blue pills, women have their little blue tubs. It is soothing, offers wonderful moisture, and has no fragrance or taste, which makes it an appealing lubricant to use during intercourse. However, you cannot use vegetable oil-based lubricants like Crisco if you are using condoms, because they break them down. Speaking of vegetable oil, if you are not a fan of Crisco, you can also use olive oil (whether or not it's extra virgin is up to you), almond oil, coconut oil, evening primrose oil, or any others. The secret is to make sure you have *something* down there at all times.

When it comes to making love, you may want to step up to the sexual lubricants that last longer, are less messy, and do not break down condoms like some of the vegetable oils do. There are water-based and non-water-based jellies, liquids, and gels. Astro-Glide seems to always rate the highest among women. One of the newer ones that is gaining in popularity is called Pjur and is made in Germany. It is not water-based like most others tend to be, and it lasts a long time without any stickiness or need to reapply. If you have a good adult store near you—one that also caters to gay men—you will find a large selection from which to choose.

Approach the need to enhance your sex life through the use of lubricants with a sense of adventure, not shame or shyness. Yes, you have had breast cancer and you cannot change the past. But there is a future for you, and sex should be a large part of that. You don't have to stop having sex because you have atrophy and dryness due to cancer and its treatments. Utilize what is available to make things happen for you in a positive way.

You don't have to get technical with your man for the reasons you may need lubrication. Simply set it up as part of the wonderful lovemaking experience. It is all in how you present it. If you are nervous and embarrassed, he will pick up on it. But if you are excited and offering it as part of the evening's fun, he will love it. Do your best to relax and enjoy lubricants. You can be more discreet and pre-apply a lubricant that comes in a bead, like KY Liquibeads, so you don't have to stop during lovemaking, or you can make it part of the experience by having him put them on you. Arrange them next to the bed on a pretty tray with a flower. Make it exciting . . . because it is!

Vaginal Atrophy

Vaginal atrophy is the thinning and tightening of the vagina, and it often accompanies dryness. Over time, atrophy can tighten the first third of your vagina so much that any sex is painful. It can even progress to the point where it becomes a problem to wear certain clothes, like jeans, or to enjoy certain activities, like exercise, because the vaginal tissues have become thin to the point that they get abraded and raw.

Did you ever think about vaginal atrophy before cancer? Should any woman ever have to worry about this horror? Um, *no!* Unfortunately, because of your cancer and treatments, you will need to become aware of it. It may creep up on you, especially if you are doing a long run of chemo. But as soon as you notice something is happening down there, get to work.

Keep It Busy

The vaginal walls supply lubrication. With proper stimulation—keeping it busy—you can increase the blood supply to the tissues. This will not only increase lubrication, but it will also increase the elasticity of the vagina, which will help improve atrophy. In other words, if you maintain a good and active blood supply to your vagina on a regular basis, you can prevent or reverse dryness and atrophy. Remember, though, that there are all levels of atrophy. Hopefully stimulation will prevent it completely. But if it has already started, get busy and stop it.

On top of using stimulation, you can also manually improve atrophy by lubricating your fingers and inserting them into your vagina once a day. This will gently stretch the area a little bit at a time. It may seem like a simple solution, and if you do it in combination with stimulation, these simple measures can reverse atrophy and bring you back to your old self again.

Topical Estrogen

Some women's atrophy is so severe that simple stimulation alone won't help. They are in so much pain that even urinating hurts. When this is the case, almost all gynecologists want to prescribe topical estrogen. However, if these women had estrogen-sensitive cancer, almost all oncologists tell them they are forbidden to use it. This is because oncologists feel that adding exogenous estrogen will blunt the effects of endocrine therapy, thereby increasing chances of recurrence.

Where oncologists are charged with saving lives, gynecologists are all about improving the quality of lives. And, in this instance, the gynecological argument is compelling. Many gynecologists claim that the level of topical estradiol is so low that the small amount absorbed by the body won't make a systematic difference. Therefore, they often do a baseline estradiol test when they start therapy, and then, three months later, do another serum-level test to see if it has spiked. Almost all women have no significant increase. If they do, therapy is either stopped or reduced. But by then, the estrogen has already done the trick and the woman is well on her way to feeling human again.

Again, the systemic absorption risk is very low. Consider this comparison: A low dose hormone replacement therapy pill that you ingest has 1,000 micrograms of estradiol, whereas the topically insertable vaginal tablet only has 25 micrograms of estradiol. This should give you an idea of how little estrogen these topical treatments expose you to, and how absorption into the bloodstream is almost non-existent. This small to almost non-existent risk is, in many women's opinion, greatly outweighed by the improved quality of life from the little bit that is applied to the irritated tissues.

If your gynecologist recomends a topical estrogen treatment for your atrophy, which one should you choose? There are vaginal creams, as well as dissolvable vaginal tablets that can be inserted. The creams can be messy and harder to calibrate than the tablets. But you also have more control over them, which can be comforting. Just a small dot of cream applied around the labia and the vulva can bring big relief. Finally, know that the use of these topical agents does not have to be long term. Once you get your body back and your skin is once again supple, you can ditch the creams and tablets for the natural route of moisturizers and stimulation.

Non-Estrogen Based Topical Therapy

If you want to err on the side of caution and not introduce estrogen into your body at all, you might want to try a product called Replens. It has been proven to increase lubrication, heal atrophied vaginal tissues, and improve women's dryness problems. It comes in a tube from which you insert the product vaginally every three days. When you first start using it you will have a white discharge similar to that which comes with a yeast infection. This is normal. It is a culmination of the dead skin cells that line the vaginal walls. They are being shed to make way for fresh, supple tissue underneath, which, by definition, is the reversal of atrophy.

Topical testosterone is another non-estrogen choice for women to treat atrophy and dryness. Although this is fairly new and studies are still ongoing, it appears that topical testosterone can help reverse atrophy almost as well as topical estrogen. This is something that you should discuss with your doctor as a potential option for you to use.

TOY STORY

Now that you know how important vaginal stimulation is, you're probably wondering how exactly to go about doing it. These days, sex toys are officially out of the closet (or drawer) and they are everywhere. Many women openly admit to owning at least one vibrator. However, many others have no idea what to buy, where to begin, or why they even need toys, because sex was always good enough without them. Sex aside, if you use toys a minimum of three times a week, you can reverse your dryness and atrophy, increase your libido, and learn about your new body—something you can eventually share with your partner.

If you are suffering from severe atrophy, your gynecologist has medical toys that can get you started. They come in the form of graduated, vibrating dilators. They start small. Then, as you get used to the first size, you move on to the next. You keep moving on until the blood supply to your vagina has increased enough for it to do its magic with the elasticity of your vaginal walls. Soon after learning with these medical toys, you can graduate to the adult toy store.

Have you ever been to a sex toy shop? Are you too embarrassed to go to one in person? If so, you can always order items from the Internet or a catalog. However, you can get a better idea of size and function in person. Look for a variety of items including things that vibrate for pleasure and increased blood flow, as well as things that can be inserted to start opening you up again. In a sex toy store, you will see all kinds of toys in every size imaginable, and in every color of the rainbow.

One of the bestselling toys is the Hitachi Massager—also known in some quarters as "Mr. Big." You can get attachments to go with it that will do just about anything you want. There are also imaginative items that are built for simultaneous insertion and stimulation. These usually have some type of animal attached to them, like a rabbit, to provide clitoral stimulation, as well as insertable swirling pearls that are meant to target the G-Spot. In addition, these swirling pearls do a wonderful job of opening you up and increasing blood flow.

Here is a brief breakdown of the different types of toys that you can buy:

Massagers

Yes, your grandmother had one, and no, it wasn't used for her rheumatism! Massagers are sold everywhere and are typically marketed on their packages as providing "deep, soothing pain relief." The head of a massager is usually soft and rounded, and it vibrates with a flip of a switch at the base. It can be used on your neck, lower back, and other areas. The fun starts when it's used for the "other areas." These days, massagers are high-tech and come with all sorts of things you can add on to them. You can even purchase a basic model at your local drugstore. At the checkout counter, rub your neck and also buy Bengay if you are worried and embarrassed that the pharmacist is on to you. Chances are, though, there is one in her bedroom drawer, too!

Vibrators

Vibrators do one thing: vibrate. They don't pretend to be massagers, they are quick and to the point, and they can be purchased online or at adult toy stores. Vibrators come in many shapes and sizes, and can even be as small as a lipstick tube. In fact, some are disguised to look like lipstick. Others are designed to look like loofah sponges or rubber duckies. If you are musically inclined, there are vibrators that can be attached to your iPod that work with your favorite, feel-good songs. There are even disposable vibrators that come with condoms. They aren't a big investment, and you throw them out when the batteries die. These disguised items might be a good option for you if you are uncomfortable with keeping sex toys in your home, for fear of someone finding them. But remember: If you don't keep your now estrogen-deprived private parts stimulated and the blood flowing down to that region, you risk pain during intercourse and the dreaded vaginal atrophy. So, get over your mortification. Really.

Dildos

Dildos are designed in the shape of a man's penis. They may or may not vibrate, and are meant for insertion. Some are large, some move, and some even have little plastic animals attached to them. They come in all sizes, shapes, and colors, and they are capable of performing all sorts of pleasures. Dildos often have cute names and can be quite expensive. But remember, you get what you pay for. Napoleon Bonaparte once said, "If you are going to take Vienna, *take* Vienna." So what the hell; if you got up the nerve to order a dildo, you might as well get the best one you can find, right? Besides, buying a quality item means it will last longer, and you won't have to order one again for a long time. Dildos can be found online, but it is best to go to a sex toy shop and look at what you are buying in real life, first. Looks can be deceiving in online photos, and it's important to make sure you are buying something that you can, um, handle.

PERSONAL STORY: JULIE'S BUDDY SYSTEM

Julie has developed a buddy system with her friend Kim, so that they can both keep their sex toys safe and secret. As she puts it, "Kim and I have made a pact. If one of us gets hit by Skylab and becomes comatose, the other is to go to our house before our family gets there to sort things out, and remove the 'goodie bag.' Kim knows exactly where mine is and I know precisely where she keeps hers. But just in case, I also have a note in my sex-toy bag that says, 'If you found this, I want you to know I am not a pervert. I need these items to keep my mojo because of breast cancer. Please put this back where you found it and move along.'"

PERSONAL STORY:
WHERE THE WILD THINGS ARE

After breast cancer treatment, you discover that vaginal dryness and atrophy are not urban legends. They can happen no matter how young you are or what your interest in sex was pre-cancer. Add hot flashes to that and you feel pretty bad when you should be feeling great.

I was in the midst of worrying about this when a friend told me that there was a place—an *adult* place—I could go to get items to prevent these things from happening to me. I had also heard that orgasms help control hot flashes. Since I was looking for assistance with both problems, I decided to give sex toys a try.

As a result, for the first time in my life, I drove to an adult toy store and forced myself to get out of the car. I was more than a little apprehensive. The windows were all covered so no one could see inside. When I walked in, I was greeted by magic crystals, patchouli incense, dragon statues, and occult looking jewelry. However, they did have very pretty sundresses on sale. I saw a sign that said, "If you want to go downstairs, you must have your ID. If you don't have your ID, then don't go downstairs."

I went downstairs. God help me.

Behind a frosted glass door, there was a selection of bongs and rolling papers, as well as an assortment of men's body parts hanging from the wall. The body parts were anatomically correct, but they came in colors—many different, bright colors. They looked like they were designed by Walt Disney.

In addition to the colorful wall decor, there were DVDs, massage oils, leather masks and leashes, objects men could wear to brighten their mood, toys that had suction cups attached to them for those times when you have the uncontrollable urge to get to know your shower wall better, and items that had things attached to them that looked like animals. At the time, I had no idea how they worked or where the animal was meant to go. And I was certainly not going to ask the fourteen-year-old cashier, particularly after the look he gave me when I asked him what the object shaped like a forearm with a clenched fist was. It looked like it fell off a Halloween display. I honestly believed it was a misplaced item from another part of the store when I held it up and asked the boy about it. I was wrong. It was in the right place. Then, to my horror, I stumbled upon the "discount bin," which was a wooden container full of sale items that had been opened or returned. The mind reels when one imagines where they have been . . .

It was then I decided I belonged upstairs with the patchouli and I made only one purchase in the Adult Toy Store: A very pretty, black and white, empire-waisted sundress.

When I got home and reported to my friend what I had purchased and what I had *not* purchased, she urged me to return. Two weeks later, I did. A different salesperson helped me this time. First he showed me an item that was a pretty shade of purple with a cute bear attached. I wasn't entirely sure what the bear was for, nor was I clear about the purpose of the metal beads inside of it that swirled like a barber shop sign. It seemed way too complicated and advanced for me, so I opted for a sleeker, simpler, more mainstream item instead.

I paid in cash, explaining to the salesperson that it wasn't for me; it was a gag gift for a bridal shower I was attending. He just smiled and said most women say the same thing. After he said that, I got over my embarrassment and out of curiosity, asked him to explain to me how the purple thing with the bear on it worked. Calmly and quietly, as if he was giving me directions to the nearest gas station, he told me. I said I would think about it for the next time and then left. I had survived making a purchase in an adult toy store. I also seriously considered returning one day for the little purple bear. . . .

7

$\mathcal{T}$he Married Survivor

The day you were diagnosed, your whole family was diagnosed. The news of your cancer impacted them, too. Not only did you have to handle that news yourself, but you had to be the one to set the tone for the entire household, which was a seemingly impossible feat to accomplish when your whole world felt like it was falling apart. You probably felt guilty, too. We women are so very hard on ourselves, aren't we? Well, you know what? Stop feeling guilty. After all, you didn't *choose* to have this disease. You didn't order it on eBay. This disease happened *to* you. Just because your entire family felt its effects, doesn't mean it's your fault. You hate it as much as they do.

YOUR HUSBAND

Hopefully, your husband honored your fight against cancer and helped you when you needed it the most, even though he was undoubtedly terrified. He may not have expressed it, but he was. And even though he has the healthy you back now, you're different. The treatments, surgeries, and fear you survived changed you, and you are just beginning to open your arms to life again. Loving husbands are often awestruck by this, but a bit intimidated, too, so be prepared. One thing that's for sure is that he *wants* you again—wants you the way you used to be. You have a chance now to show him that not only are you back, but that your family, your marital relationship, and even your love life will all be better now. After all you have been through, however, it is natural to be afraid to move forward. Acknowledge that fear, but then keep moving forward anyway. Only then will you and your husband be able to rediscover your love and passion for one another. As with everything else, it won't happen overnight or by magic. But if you take the time and make the investment in each other, you can both put cancer behind you and welcome your new life together as a team.

Recognize His Feelings

Your husband's world was rocked by your breast cancer. Not only was he worried about you during your treatments and surgeries, he was at a complete loss as to how to act around you. Now, the same thing is happening to him all over again. You are out of treatment and life is supposed to once again be normal. However, if he acts worried, he's afraid he will frighten you. If he tries to play it cool, he's worried you will think he doesn't care or isn't taking this seriously enough. And what makes this whole thing worse is that he feels like he can't help you.

Men, by nature, are doers. They like to be in action mode, not to sit on the sidelines. But when it comes to breast cancer, there's little they can do to help. There's no ladder to get, no pipe to replace, and no carburetor to fix. You would most likely be overjoyed if your husband simply took care of the laundry, but that's not what he had in mind while you were undergoing your treatment. He wished he could go to a lab somewhere and find you a cure or something, *anything*.

Now that you have begun the healing process, he wants to reassure you, but he is helpless and in uncharted waters. And men don't do helpless all that well. He doesn't know what is supposed to happen now, so he can't offer anything. Because of that, he may be hurting badly. He may also be downright mad. Just like you, he didn't plan for this. Cancer was not on his agenda, either. He won't admit it, but there were almost certainly plenty of times he asked himself, "Why isn't Harry's wife going through this instead?!"

All of these are normal emotions for a man to feel. The most important thing for you is to not let how this is affecting him, affect you. You have enough on your plate. You have to work through your own grief and healing. However, if you show him that you are capable of moving forward, that this was not some insane lifestyle choice you made, you will set a positive tone. Once you both honestly recognize that this unwelcome visitor in your lives has left the building, you can begin to work things out. Yes, the SOB known as cancer left a bit of a mess that needs to be straightened out, but together you can rebuild your lives.

Communicate

As with everything in this life, communication is key. In order to heal, you need to be able to verbalize what is happening to you physically and emotionally, and so does your husband. If both of you are talking, you will have a beautiful, albeit sometimes tough, duet. However, if just one of you is talking, you will only have a solo, which won't necessarily be listened to.

You probably want to tell your husband all about your new body, and there is a temptation to go into great detail. After all, he can likely recite your pathology report by heart, so what is so different about this? Before you spill all, though, consider your sex life. By maintaining some air of mystery and privacy, you will feel less vulnerable, while simultaneously peaking his curiosity and encouraging him to explore.

Make him aware that you are having problems, but tell him you are working on correcting them. Then, once you get into the groove of exploring your new body and feel comfortable with it, you can share those things with him. But don't say or do anything before you are ready, or before he is capable of hearing it.

Transition from Need to Want

For many months, you *needed* your husband. You needed him to drive you to doctors' appointments, to fetch your meds, to take over your part of the routine with the kids when you were too sick to deal with them, and to be strong for both of you. Now that you're recovering, you have the opportunity to make a tectonic shift in your relationship that will change things for the better, forever. It will right the ship you are on and put it back on course. Make the switch from *need* to *want*. It is that simple. Tell your husband you *want* him. That one, simple, little word will make all the difference in his world.

You may still be afraid of your new body, but guess what? So is he. Not for the same reasons you are, though. You are afraid he won't like it, that he will compare it to your pre-cancer body, or worse, that he will compare it to someone else's body. You also don't know how it works yet, and that unknown is hard to overcome.

He, on the other hand, will be afraid of hurting you. He doesn't know what or where to touch, or if you will feel pain. So reassure him. Make him feel desirable again. Tell him that you are afraid of how everything will work with this new body of yours, but you want him so much that you can't wait to figure things out together. Show him where you like to be touched and tell him to help you find new places of pleasure. Ask him if he still likes to be touched where he always did, or whether he'd like you to try some new moves. You can be like young lovers again, learning each other's bodies for the very first time. Nothing was more erotic than that, remember? You have that chance again. Embrace it. Run with it. Glory in it.

Make your first real time together, post-cancer, unforgettable. Ship the kids off somewhere, or better yet, go somewhere as a couple. Bring all your "supplies," which we will cover later, and take your husband back. Fire him as your caretaker/car driver/waiting-room-chair-warmer/worrier-in-chief, and hire him as your lover and fellow traveler on a new journey of health, love, and life.

CANCER IS EASY, MARRIAGE IS WORK

Have you ever noticed that all storybooks end with a wedding? The prince finds his princess and they live "happily ever after . . ." Really? That's all there is to it? The ring is on her finger so she doesn't have to work at her marriage or worry about a gray day anymore?

You know this isn't true. Even healthy marriages have stresses and go through many tests. The breast cancer battle certainly ranks among the toughest of these. Many marriages suffer, and some even end, when the woman gets cancer. It is hard to fathom that a man would leave his wife when she is sick. After all, most women wouldn't do that to their husbands if the situation was reversed. But it happens. So, how do we fix that and prevent it from happening to us?

For starters, we can try a little harder to take care of ourselves and to make our husbands feel like we are in this fight together. One of the men interviewed for this book had an interesting take on this concept. He has a great marriage with his wife, despite all of the struggles they have endured together. When asked what the secret to his great marriage is, his answer was simple, "She's not my wife, she's my girlfriend and she always will be."

One of the worst things that can happen in any marriage is when the couple begins taking each other and the relationship for granted. They become settled into their husband and wife roles and forget who they were when they met. The very best marriages have retained one essential key to success: The husband and wife still think of each other as they did when they dated.

When you were dating your husband, did you make sure you looked great? Or, did you open the door in baggy sweatpants with your hair all ratty and no makeup on? Now that you have a ring on your finger, do you think that it no longer matters what you look like in front of your husband? Donna Reed may have vacuumed in pearls and pumps, but her husband always saw her looking her best.

Post-cancer body issues make us hyper self-conscious. Don't make your self esteem worse by not caring what you look like anymore. Instead, remember who you and your husband were and what you meant to each other before the wedding. Quite simply: Don't stop being your husband's lover and all that it implies—excitement, mystery, passion, and above all, desire. When a man's "wife" is waiting for him at home, it implies the same old routine. But if you can somehow remain his "lover," you will keep the relationship playful and light, like it was in the beginning. Breast cancer put a damper on your marriage, but you now have a chance to rev up those old feelings again. A new you, with a new outlook on life and new things you want to try in the bedroom, will excite the brain and signal it to release dopamine and oxytocin—the chemicals that gave you a rush when you first fell in love.

In short, give yourself a "do-over." Change the way you dress and take care of yourself. Look good for *you* and he will notice. That is really the point of those lyrics. If you start to make yourself feel pretty again, to make yourself feel *good* again, you will lift both you and your husband out of Cancerland and bring joy back to your lives. If you feel good, it shows. So, if putting on a little lipstick or combing your hair makes you feel better, do it. By making these small changes, he will once again begin to see you as his lover, rather than his wife with breast cancer. But you have to make the change in you—and for you—first. Don't look outwardly for others to decide how you should act and feel about yourself. Instead, make bold moves as you are ready, and your husband will be excited by this new woman in you.

MARITAL ROUGH SPOTS

Some marriages hit rocky spots when breast cancer enters the picture. This is not abnormal. But if you see that you and your husband are heading for trouble, get help. Not later, but *now*. Communication is key. Get to the bottom of what is wrong and you may discover that it will be quite easy to fix.

Men and women often see things differently. The men that were interviewed for this book reported several things that concern and frustrate them about their wives' perceptions of themselves, their marriage, and their lives, post-cancer. Here we break down how men see some of these things, and then work out how they coincide with what may be happening with their wives. Can you see yourself in any of these real-life scenarios? Can you see how you can change things once you see them from a different point of view?

- *His Concern:* I don't know what I can do for my wife. She keeps saying she is ugly. I think she looks great. I don't care about the scars, but she keeps pushing it so every conversation revolves around her telling me how unattractive she thinks she is, and me trying to talk her out of it.

Your Turn: Are you harping about your looks? Do you feel insecure to the point that you have gone blind to how beautiful you really are? How bad is it? If you are really that down on yourself, get to a counselor and get some therapy. But first, take a look at the chapter on beauty (page 41) and try some, or all, of the ideas discussed in it. Then revisit this question.

- *His Concern:* I don't feel like I matter anymore. She is all-consumed in cancer. I thought once she was done with everything she would lighten up, but she seems more consumed now than when she was sick.

Your Turn: The fact that you are all-consumed with cancer is normal. It is a process that you have to work through. Eventually, as your calendar clears up and there are fewer doctor appointments, you will see that you have more time for fun things and that you can breathe again. However, if fear is interfering with your daily life, you may need counseling. Ask yourself how you want to live the life you have fought so hard for. Take a look at Chapter 13 (page 169). It may help you see things differently.

- *His Concern:* She doesn't want to do anything anymore and she hates it when I talk about the future. She always has to say, "Well I won't be around then." The doctor says she is going to be around a long time, but she doesn't believe him.

Your Turn: Are you suffering from the "other shoe syndrome"? Do you fear that when you put away your winter clothes for the summer, you may never see them again because you won't survive until Labor Day? Accept your disease. You had it. Acknowledge what you did to fight it. Did you fight it with everything you had? Did you do everything they told you to? Is there anything more they said you needed to do that you are not doing? If so, do it. If not, move forward and don't look back. Live for today, not for what *may* happen, because you rob yourself of life's joys if you don't.

- *His Concern:* No matter how hard I try, I can't seem to make her happy anymore.

  Your Turn: Are you that unhappy? If you find yourself truly sad every day, if you sleep more than usual or don't seem to sleep at all, if you have no interest in daily activities, or if you have feelings of hopelessness and feel like a dark hole in the world is swallowing you up, you may be clinically and chemically depressed. Depression is as real an illness as any other, and it is not unusual for it to happen after cancer. Your brain chemicals are altered and you may need an antidepressant. Get help. You can turn this around. You can end the depression and start living again. See Chapter 13 (page 169).

- *His Concern:* She doesn't like sex anymore. I feel like a pervert now if I attempt to get close to her.

  Your Turn: You may not like sex anymore because it hurts. This book shows you how to get your body back to enjoying sex again, though. Your libido may also be lacking. If it is, check out the medications you are on. They could be at fault. Certain antidepressants can turn off your libido. but there are others that do not have that side effect. Speak to your doctor and switch. Don't let your husband feel like a pervert. Get to know your body again and show him some new moves.

EVEN GOOD MARRIAGES CAN SUFFER

There are some men that just cannot cope with the enormity of cancer. It is a sad fact that sometimes the one person you thought you could lean on the most, turns out to be the last person you can turn to when you're in need. It is hard to imagine a husband not being there for his wife, but some simply cannot handle having their wives sick and out of commission, or the extra burden that it may put on them. These men are especially sensitive to the fact that they feel like everyone is watching them to see how they'll handle your time of need. They feel like everyone expects them to be great husbands, which is a hard image to live up to if it's simply not in them.

You've got to remember that you can't change people. We are all wired differently, and we are either equipped to handle the good along with the bad, or we are not. Your husband may stand by you, or he may become distant. He may feel incredible empathy and compassion toward you, or he may be overcome with the enormity of it all. However he feels, it is *his* problem—it is most definitely not yours.

You must focus on getting your own life back. Never underestimate how capable, strong, and self-sufficient you are. But also, never underestimate the need for help. If your marriage is in trouble and you think it is worth saving, then get both your butts into counseling. You may find out a lot about each other that you held in the entire time you were in treatment, and it may help. Be aware, though, that you may find out things you don't want to hear, too. It is all part of therapy.

When Counseling Should Be Considered

If you are having marital problems, you will know it. But to what degree do you let it get before you suggest help? If there is no communication at all, if you feel like you are living with a stranger, if he has no interest in you, your health, your victories, or your fears, then that is more than enough of a warning sign. If you want to fight for your marriage now that you are done fighting your cancer, then get counseling or therapy of some sort. Chances are, that is the only way you will work things out.

Find a therapist for yourself first. Learn how to recognize your feelings, and also how to vocalize them to your husband. You have to heal personally, as well as heal as a couple. When you and your therapist think it is time, get your husband into therapy, too. The best option is to have him get individual therapy, too, and then combine that with couple therapy. After all, he also has things he needs to work out, and he may not want to do so in front of you.

How to Find a Good Therapist

Your oncologist's office should have resources that contain information about local psychologists, psychiatrists, therapists, and counselors who specialize in couples affected by cancer. If you can't find help there, though, try your other doctors. Your breast surgeon, your reconstructive surgeon, or even your gynecologist may have some names of good people. If you're still striking out, the American Cancer Society, local community groups, faith-based programs, and word of mouth can also help.

What you need is someone with whom you and your husband both feel comfortable. You need someone that your husband will open up to and want to talk to. If he is bucking the process because he hates the doctor, you are wasting your time. But if you can get him to therapy and you can talk this out, you may be able to save your marriage. Sometimes, though, it just doesn't work out. That is another reason you need individual therapy. It can help you if you have to take a step in a direction that is very painful.

WHEN TO CUT YOUR LOSSES AND START OVER

If you've tried therapy and your marriage is still rocky, it's time to be brutally honest with yourself. Did you fight cancer to live a life of misery with a man who does not appreciate or love you anymore? Is it worth staying with someone simply because you've always been together and know nothing else? Is making another life-altering change after what you just went through out of the question right now?

Only you know the answers to these questions. It is your life ahead of you. You've got to choose how you want to live it, and how you want to enjoy it. Think long and carefully—this is not a small decision and it should not be taken lightly. Starting over is scary, but it can also be exhilarating. Cancer has a way of opening the windows and blowing all the chaff out of our lives. That can be a very good thing. And it can also be as scary as hell.

First and foremost, you need to protect yourself if you are considering this move. If you are on his health insurance policy, you need to work that into the settlement or sign up for an individual plan within the same company. You cannot be denied coverage for a pre-existing condition if you are just switching plans with your same provider. You also need to assess where you are in combined debt.

Whose name is the house in? Do you have joint credit cards? If so, immediately get your name off of all of them and start establishing your own, personal credit history. This can be done small at first. Open an account, buy a few things, and then pay off the bill in full as soon as you receive it.

Similarly, if you have a joint bank account, the first thing you need to do is open your own account. If you are still in the planning stages of ending your marriage, do this privately. Get a post office box and have the statements sent there. Use a new bank, not the one where you have your joint account. Then, start filling that new account slowly so you have a nest egg to rely on when your marriage really does end.

When you are close to telling your husband that it's over between the two of you, go see a lawyer first. Some marriages can end in a collaborative manner with one shared attorney. However, that may not work for you. Do not share a lawyer if you have a lot of assets. Your lawyer will direct you in what you need to do legally to move forward. But at least you will have already done the preliminary work to protect yourself, your finances, and your credit history.

PERSONAL STORY: WHEN AMY ACCEPTED THAT HER MARRIAGE WAS OVER

My story is simple. When the doctors discovered my cancer, my husband Jim wanted nothing to do with it. He would complain to me that I was lying around on the sofa too much, and that I was getting fat. He would also leave our boys with me and go fishing for the weekend, even on my bad days after chemo. It was hard to take care of a five- and seven-year-old when I felt so miserable.

When my treatments were over, Jim expected me to bounce right back. But I couldn't. Part of the problem was the chemo side effects, but the other was what I thought was depression. I was getting worse instead of better. I didn't feel like leaving the house and I barely took care of myself, much less my sons. When I had a follow-up appointment at my oncologist's office, I asked him for sleeping pills. He asked me how much sleep I had been getting on average, so I told him I didn't sleep at night, but I did a lot during the day. This brought on a lot more questions from him. Finally, he strongly suggested that I see a psychologist.

Jim was dead against it, but I went anyway. And what I learned was that I was not really depressed, I was furious. I guess I had been holding in all the anger I felt toward Jim and the way he treated me, because I felt so weak and helpless when I was sick. After this realization, I told Jim that I wanted him to get therapy, too. He refused, and there was no way I was going to change his mind. He still blamed me for everything and said nothing he did needed to be "talked" about.

A few months later, I needed another surgery. It was an emergency gallbladder surgery and I was in a lot of pain. Jim, however, was "too busy" to take me to the hospital, so I wound up taking a cab. I was in the hospital for a week. He only came to see me twice.

When I got better, I told him that he either needed to get therapy, or that I would leave. I have no idea where that came from inside of me, but I did know that I wanted a better life for myself. And I also did not want my sons to grow up with him as an example of how a man should act.

Jim refused to go, of course, so I went to a lawyer and started proceedings. We are divorced now, and I am in love with a new, wonderful man who thinks I am wonderful, too. I had never felt cherished before, but now I do. My boys love him. Trevor, the oldest, said to me that he loves Michael because "he made his mommy happy for the first time."

Jim is alone now. I feel sorry for him. But I feel great for myself. I feel like I am soaring. I got rid of two toxic things in my life at one time—cancer and Jim. It feels great.

8

Sex and the Married Survivor

You don't feel like the same woman you were when you were first married, or when you were first diagnosed. And you aren't! You are so much more. Don't wait to see what your husband's reaction to the post-treatment you is to define yourself. You decide. Be your own woman. Your recent fight against cancer has taught you a lot about what you are made of. There is a fire in you now, and you have a new perspective on life that you never had before. This perspective also applies to how you view yourself and how you project your self image.

Once you feel like you know who you are again, re-introduce yourself to your husband. If your battle changed you from Amiable Amy to Hurricane Helen, he is going to have to adjust a bit. Be true to yourself, but also cut the guy a break. This is all new to him. Dialogue is the best medicine, so do your best to get everything out in the open. Tell him, hey, I know I have changed. But change doesn't have to be bad—it can be for the better. Only when you both become comfortable with the new you will your sex life once again flourish.

PROJECT CONFIDENCE

If you feel insecure or like damaged goods, it will emanate from you like a dense fog. How you carry yourself goes a long way in determining how people perceive you. There are drop-dead gorgeous women who have no self-confidence, and they make themselves less attractive because of it. Conversely, there are butt-ugly women who act like they are the stunningly beautiful; they announce to anyone within earshot how "hot" and "awesome" they are, and people start to believe it. It's amazing. Imagine the results if a beautiful woman, if *you*, did that?

Every morning when you get up, look at yourself in the mirror and say, "I am beautiful." Yes, you have probably heard it before. But have you ever tried it? Have you ever done it every single day? Do it religiously for a month, and then decide if it is a cliché.

Even when you feel your worst, put on some makeup, stand up straight, and walk confidently into any situation. Maybe you don't look your best that day, but remind yourself that even though your hair may look like crap, you have a stunning immune system. You do! You beat cancer with that immune system and that is not nothing. Get yourself thinking positively in any way you can and it will radiate from you. People will be so impressed that they won't notice anything else.

REDISCOVER YOUR MOJO

A dirty mind is a terrible thing to waste. You used to think about things like pleasure and desire, but recently you have been preoccupied with things like pathology reports and your toenails falling off. Really hot, huh? Get your head out of Cancerland! Refocus it on your sexuality. Watch some romantic movies—and even some more-than-romantic movies—that will visually remind you of just how much fun sex is. Play the rock songs that you used to play when getting ready to go clubbing twenty years ago. Do whatever it takes to once again get your mind thinking sexy thoughts.

Then, schedule a real date with your husband. Take your time getting ready for it and make yourself as gorgeous as you can. Don't stop at just a little mascara and lip-gloss. Go all out with your hair and makeup—the kind of getting ready for an important date that you used to do. The whole idea is to get your mind back in the land of the loving. And the only way to do that is to completely and utterly let go of everything that has to do with cancer. Look inside yourself and ask that amazing woman to come back out and stay there.

When you have your date, take it slow. Let your husband compliment you, and more importantly, believe him when he does. Make out with him on the sofa and slowly build up your repertoire. When you feel your husband become aroused, ask yourself who got him there. *You* did. Tell yourself over and over that he wants *you*. Honey, they removed your breasts, not your DNA. You are still a woman—then, now, and always. You still smell great. Your neck still tastes sweet. Your soft sighs as your husband kisses you still come totally and completely from your female chromosomes. Stick with it until you find your mojo again. Sink back into your femininity. Surrender to seduction and allow yourself to feel all the delicious feelings you have missed for so long. Say hello to the woman in you. She is still there and she is waiting for you.

COMMUNICATE

There are all kinds of men and all kinds of women. Rarely are any of them on the same wavelength, even in the best of conditions. Therefore, you and your husband's timing, post-treatment, may be light years apart. *You* may be ready for the reveal. *You* may be ready to show him your new body. But he may not be ready to see it.

The reason for this is not that he doesn't love you. It is because he, too, has been through an emotional upheaval. He has been worried about you, more so than he could ever let on. While you were freaking out about losing your hair, he was freaking out about losing you. Now it's all over. The doctors have given you the green light to move forward with your lives, and you have been watching yourself heal. The disconnect between you and your new body has been lessened, and you are starting to feel more as one with yourself. However, your husband still has a lot of connecting to do.

First, he must stand down. You are asking him to come out and play, but he is still looking for enemy troops lurking in the bushes, coming to take you away from him again. Since you are no longer on

Defcon1, tell him that his armor can be put away. In addition, he may just not be ready to see your breasts. That doesn't mean he doesn't want to make love to you. In fact, he never stopped wanting to make love to you. Most often, the reason that men hold back is because they don't want to appear callous by requesting a romp in the hay too soon after your battle. Thus, it's your job to make him understand that there are no more infusions and that there is no more fighting to do.

Furthermore, you have to get your timing in sync. To do that, you need to *talk*. Talk about what you want to do with him. Talk about what you feel comfortable showing him right now. Then ask him what he feels comfortable seeing. If he shrinks back from your offer to let him see you naked, it is not necessarily because it will turn him off. Most likely, it is because it will be a psychological flashback for him. It will remind him of the fear and pain he experienced while watching you endure all that you did. If this is the case with you and your partner, suggest making love with a t-shirt on, or better yet, while wearing one of his button-down shirts—there is nothing sexier! If your breasts are covered, it will seem to him like nothing happened to you—like you jumped in a time machine and he has you back from before all that you, as a team, went through.

Once you reconnect and rediscover that intimacy, you will most likely find that you are both ready to expose yourselves. Your part is easy. All you have to do is take off your shirt. His part is harder, though, because he will have to open up to you about just how scared and vulnerable he was when you were ill. Let him share that with you. Then, once the words are out there, the healing can begin and the loving can get better.

NEW SEX—
IT'S NOT THE WAY IT USED TO BE, IT'S BETTER

Men are pretty simple creatures, but when it comes to post-treatment sex you can bet that your husband is just as nervous as you are. He has seen how much pain you have been in. He has seen you sick, weak, and struggling. However, he has also seen you emerge from that. You are now well. It is true that you may have lingering side effects from medications that you must take forever to keep the cancer away. But your hair is back and your reconstruction, if you had it, is complete.

Your husband used to have a sexual repertoire. He knew how to touch you and what pleased you. But now when he looks at your beautiful, new breasts they stare back at him and seem to say, "Okay fella, show me what you got." He quite simply does not know how or where to touch you anymore. He doesn't know how to make love to you. After all, if you, the owner of this new body, don't know how it works and what to do with it, how confused do you think your husband is? Pretty stumped! He is afraid he may hurt you. He is afraid you may see something in his face that will make you think he doesn't find you as desirable as ever, so he ends up making weird faces that make you even more concerned. The guy is a mess.

You have to take over. Teach him about your new body. Show him what you have learned in your latest explorations and make it as exciting and enticing as you can. There are no wrong moves or wrong touches. Let him explore and as he does, gently correct him. Or better yet, move his hand to where you want it to be without saying a word. Touch him in new ways, too. Surprise him. If your old sex routine was just that, a routine, shake things up a bit. Try wearing new lingerie to help set things in motion, and then keep it interesting throughout your time together. The trick is to be patient. This is all new to him, too. You have an opportunity to change things for the better and to do things together you never did before. Let him know you understand. Tell him that you are also afraid, but that together you can overcome anything.

After you have made love, focus on the positive. Right when you finish is not the time for suggestions. Wait until breakfast to discuss those. If you don't believe me, consider this: A group of married men were asked one question and given the choice of three answers. The question was, "What would you like to do the most after making love?" And the answers to choose from were, "Go to sleep," "Talk about the lovemaking," and "Eat something and watch TV." Which answer do you think received the lowest number of votes? Here is a hint: The first and last answers scored the highest. Take it from me and these men: Don't be the John Madden of the bedroom and give a halftime report and post-game analysis. Men hate to analyze sex. Make mental notes for yourself for the next time, but for now, leave the guy alone.

The bottom line is that with the changes your body has gone through and the need for certain new bedroom items, your post-treatment sex will not be the way it used to be for you two. But this does not have to be a negative thing. The words "new" and "exciting" are always good when it comes to sex. Forget about your old routine and get creative with making a new one. Show him how to use one of your toys on you or get lubrication for his pleasure, too. You know you have it in you, so have some fun!

BREAST MEN VERSUS LEG MEN

Many women classify their husbands as either "breast men" or "leg men." But what does that even mean? If you don't have great legs anymore, will your husband leave you? Probably not. Similarly, will a change in your breasts terminate your relationship? True, some men are just not very nice and marriages and relationships can end because of breast cancer. But if you have a good man and a good marriage, he can overcome his penchant for breasts and can even learn to love your new, enhanced, perky reconstructions.

There is another option if this is really worrying you. You can work on your lower body to either keep your leg-man husband happy, or to convince your breast-man husband to join the other team. Bike, swim, walk, or run—do whatever you enjoy most and get in good shape. Through this exercise, not only will you improve your physical self, but your confidence will also soar. And if you feel confident about your body, you will begin to carry yourself better, which, in itself, is a turn on.

Before you become paranoid and feel you must change your body to keep your husband happy, though, take a minute to consider the trivial nature of this notion by turning it around to women. After all, we could be similarly classified as "hair women" or "ab women."

If you are a hair woman and your husband goes bald, will you leave him? Or, if you are an ab woman and his once upon a time six-pack abs now look more like he's in the third trimester of a pregnancy, are you going to call it quits on your marriage? No. Chances are, he's not going to, either.

DEALING WITH OTHER WOMEN'S REAL BREASTS

Forget denying it. You know you look at other women's natural breasts. But why? Maybe you sneak peaks because you don't have them any-more, or maybe it's because you are comparing your new ones to other women's original ones. Regardless, it's a natural curiosity.

What's more disconcerting is that you also catch your husband checking out other women's real chests. But let's be honest here. Did he only recently start doing this? Or has he done this since he was thirteen but you are only noticing it now? Most likely, the latter is true. Many women who have battled cancer have said that they have found pictures of topless women on their husbands' comput-ers. They are shocked and hurt, and they feel betrayed. If this should happen to you, please remember that he was looking at these pic-tures long before you ever had cancer. The only difference is that now you notice it, and it makes you crazy because you have lost your breasts.

News flash! If you were photographed topless with your implants and then airbrushed, you would look just like those women. So if it really bothers you, put on some sexy panties, strike an alluring pose, set your camera's timer, and take a picture of yourself. Then, down-load it to your computer and Photoshop it to airbrush out your scars and cellulite. Make it hot! Then, send it to your husband's computer. Try it. You will make his day.

PERSONAL STORY:
CONFESSIONS OF A BREAST MAN

When guys sit around and talk about women, one question that is bound to come up is, "Are you a breast man or a leg man?" The first answer is always, "Both." Knowing that we live in reality and that we can't ask for both perfect breasts and perfect legs, though, the breakdown is always 60/40 with breasts winning out. I admit that I am a breast man. I always have been.

When I met my wife, you can be sure that her breasts were one of the first things I noticed. She had a beautiful body and a beautiful face, and she always took care of her looks. She could spend hours, yes *hours*, putting her face on. As infuriating as it could be, it was always worth it when she came strolling out of the bedroom, dressed to the nines and looking like a million bucks. I watched her body carry our three children, woke up to her gorgeous face for thirty years, and I never fell out of love with her. We have had our hard times and we fight like tigers, but we always manage to make up, eventually.

I was the one who actually found the lump in her breast. My hand passed over it and I froze. She made a doctor appointment the next morning, and our worst fear was realized. She had breast cancer. The doctors said it was big and she would most likely lose the breast. After a long talk with them, she came home and told me that she wanted both taken off.

She was worried about how I would take the news. I felt like the weight of the world was on me. Why should she start worrying about me? Everything was happening to her—not me! She was also worried about the kids. I bet if I asked her, she was probably even worried about how the mailman would take the news, too. I am not going to lie and say I wasn't devastated, and that surgery seemed so drastic that it made the cancer even scarier to me. But it was about more than just her body at that point. I was scared I was going to lose her.

Everything happens pretty fast in this. Before I could turn around, I was sitting in a pre-operating room with her holding her hand. She didn't blink when they inserted the IV. She was wearing a shower cap and a couple of cloth gowns, one facing front and one facing back. She also had on special socks with treads on the bottom. I liked those—wished I could get a pair. She rolled her eyes when I asked the nurse for some, but the nurse slipped me a size extra large anyway. I still have them.

The doctor came in and said it was time. I kissed my beautiful wife goodbye. I didn't know what our world would be like after this. I felt like I was saying goodbye to a whole chunk of our history together as lovers. She told me to stop crying and to go get something to eat. And then she walked out of the room with a doctor on one side and a nurse on the other.

Later that day, the doctor came out to tell me everything went great. He said all the cancer was removed. They had to take her lymph nodes because the test said the cancer had spread, but he said he got rid of them and all the tissue around them. He then told me it would be another hour before the plastic surgeon finished with her. They do it as a tag team. First the cancer surgeon takes off the breast and cancer, and then the plastic surgeon puts her back together again.

After awhile, I got to see my wife in the recovery room. It scared me because she looked like she had been through a lot. Her lips were swollen and puffy, and she was out of it. The nurse told me to come back in a half an hour. When I did, she was looking like her old self— well, the way she did the morning after one of our Christmas parties. She had expanders in her chest to push out her muscle in order to make room for her future implants. Funny, I was always proud that my wife never needed implants because her breasts were full and round. But that was in the past now.

She was allowed to come home two days later even though she was still in a lot of pain. She had drains hanging out of her and she didn't want me near them. She did everything that pertained to the personal care of her surgery herself, despite my numerous offers. I was allowed to help with pillows and pain pills, though, and I made sure she was eating all her favorite foods.

About a month later, after her expanders had been filled a couple of times, we were getting ready for bed when a look that I had come to know so well spread across her face. It is the look that I love—it means she wants to be close to me. However, this time I was terrified. I didn't want to hurt her. Was she still in pain? I was also scared of my reaction to her. What if my face gave away my shock? She, on the other hand, was acting like nothing had happened to her. She wanted to make love. It was like she had put her cancer experience in a box and locked it in the closet for the night.

When she took off her nightgown, I saw her new breasts for the first time. Were they the same as her old ones? No. There were scars going across them and she had no nipples. I was both shocked and fascinated at the same time. I said, "Wow." She said, "What does that mean?" And I told her, truthfully, that this reconstruction process was going to be something very interesting to watch. It was like she was being transformed back into the woman she wanted to be right before my eyes.

We made love, alright. And it was good—as good as it always was. Every time I looked at her breasts, I admit that I was a little taken aback. But that was just the first night. After that night, she started dressing in front of me and not hiding herself anymore. And I honestly got used to them. It was exciting to see how they grew every time she came home from a fill-up. This was something new to both of us.

When she started chemotherapy, she lost her hair. She never let me see her without something on her head. She either wore a scarf or one of her wigs, and she always slept in a little knit hat. But her breasts were available to me. I liked being part of that process. She always said the breasts are forever, the bald is only temporary, so she didn't want me to see that.

Fast forward to now. Her chemo and radiation are done, and her doctor said she is good to go. He feels she has every reason to believe she beat cancer. Her hair is an inch long and she dyed it bright blonde. She just had her permanent implants put in and they are so soft to the touch, not like the hard expanders. She also told me that she scheduled her nipple replacement and that she wants me there to pick the size and color.

Our sex life took a nosedive when she was in chemo. But now that she is feeling better, we have begun again. We have had to make a few adjustments here and there, but making them together seems to add to the pleasure for both of us.

I love my wife. And I love her new body even more than her old one, because this one saved her life. Her new breasts mean that her cancer is gone. They are symbols of her future and of everything positive that comes out of fighting cancer—and believe it or not, there is an awful lot of positive that comes out of that hateful disease.

Do I miss her old breasts? Yes and no. I like to think of them as a great, classic car I once owned that got totaled, but the construction of it saved the lives of the passengers inside. My wife's old breasts almost killed her. I am glad they are history. We have a shiny new model now, and while I can look back wistfully at the old classic, this new one is better and so much safer.

After all this, if I was in a locker room full of guys today and I was asked if I was a breast man or a leg man, my answer would still be: *"Hell yeah I am a breast man. My wife's new breasts are the most beautiful things I have ever seen. And they aren't even done yet."*

LET YOUR LIGHT SHINE

Look at the colors of a Tiffany lampshade. They're pretty, aren't they? The intricate scrolls of the lead between each piece of carefully selected stained glass look almost like lace. Now, turn on the light in the lamp. The lampshade comes to life and goes from nice to magnificent. Pinks, purples, and indigos bounce off of each other, filling the whole room with delicate reflections of beauty and artistry.

Your husband knows what is behind *your* lampshade. He knows the real you inside, and that is who he fell in love with. Your husband is someone with whom you have a commitment—he is not some fling that is just quickly glancing at your lampshade. He knows that it is the light within you that makes any covering blossom to life. He knows that true beauty comes from deep inside you, and that the light that is radiated from a confident, strong, effervescent woman is worth more than any reconstruction or scar you may have. In fact, your scars become part of the intricate scrolls that separate and elucidate the true, deep colors within you.

When your husband tells you he thinks you are beautiful, believe him. He has known you for a long time. He knows your light within, and he knows that there is more to you than a couple of scars. Now *you* need to believe that, too. Let your light shine brightly. He will be blinded by the colors that come off of you. The more desirable he makes you feel—that you *let* him make you feel—the brighter and deeper your colors will become. A man who loves the light inside you sees only beauty, not scars. You are rare and precious, so shine on you beautiful diamond, you.

9

$\mathcal{T}$he Single Survivor

It seems that breast cancer patients are almost always portrayed as mothers or grandmothers smiling bravely while surrounded by their beautiful children. It's a very touching image because it breaks your heart to think about the worry they must go through for their families.

But there is another type of survivor, too. She is the one who takes herself to all her treatments and has to go out and get her own ginger ale. She is young and single, and she has had breast cancer. You never hear her story, though. You never learn about how her life is completely changed forever. Cancer has devastated many of her dreams and plans in some form or another, but the pink and blue catalogs doctors dispense don't have a chapter for her. She doesn't fit in with the marketing plan.

This single survivor started her life the same way most young girls do. She played with dolls, did her homework, went to college, and started her career. She always knew she would someday meet the right man, get married, and have a family of her own. But now, she starts to doubt this. She worries that "someday" may not come.

After all the surgeries and chemo, her body is now a stranger to her. The doctors say she can live a normal life, but "normal" now may mean a life without children, and with psychological damage that has affected her body image and self-esteem. The fear of exposing this new body to a new lover is unrelenting, especially when she is just getting accustomed to it herself.

If this is you, if you are a single survivor, keep your chin up. Even though thoughts like these are uppermost in your mind right now, they don't have to be forever. The farther you get from treatments and doctor's offices, the better you will feel. And the better you feel, the closer you will be to reclaiming your life—in whatever form it may take. Unfortunately, there is no instruction manual that tells you precisely how to accomplish this. You have to find your own way, but it can be done—one step at a time.

Take back control of your life. Don't live with cancer hovering over you. You let cancer win if it still calls the shots. Also, don't let other people treat you as if you will always and forever be the girl who is living in the cancer spotlight. You may actually be guilty of this yourself if you think that is all you are now. Get rid of those thoughts. You were a fabulous woman before cancer entered your life, and you are even more magnificent now that it has been beaten back out of your life. Remember that!

DON'T ALLOW YOURSELF TO BE DIMINISHED

There is a strange phenomenon that surrounds you as a single breast cancer survivor. Some people view you as a non-person. If they have a single, male friend, they don't consider introducing you to him because you are the "Designated Cancer Patient," which apparently means you are not a woman anymore.

These same people get annoyed that you live in a house instead of an apartment. They think that there is some secret, unwritten rule that orders all single women—especially those who are cancer survivors—to be housed in garden apartments. If you dare to have a house, a yard, a garden, and even—gasp!—a picket fence, you are not living like you are on borrowed time. You are actually living and making long-term plans. In fact, you are getting very close to encroaching onto married, healthy people's territory—"their" territory. They may be offended, but who cares?

Beware of the toxic people in your life who see you as a non-entity. Don't allow anyone to diminish you or the struggles you have been through. This applies to both male and female friends who seem to have a problem with the fact that you look even better now than you did before cancer. We will pray for them later. In the meantime, let's get out the barbeque and have a few friends over, shall we?

BREAKING THE NEWS TO BOYFRIENDS

When you do start dating again—and you *will* date again—there is no right or wrong time to tell your new beau about your medical history. You have been alive for a very long time. You have accomplished a lot and you have a whole history. Cancer is only *part* of that history. It does not define you and it does not wipe out the rest of your life. It was a challenge that you took on, fought like hell, and defeated.

When you go on a dinner date, remember that the man sitting across from you is with a magnificent warrior. He is with *you*—you who has overcome so much. When you feel the time is right and the man is worthy of knowing more about you than all of the wonderful things you have already told him, you can then mention that you had cancer. In the words of Margaret Thatcher, "This is no time to go all wobbly." Keep the emphasis on the word *had*. You *had* cancer. Life is what you *have* now.

Don't be in a hurry to reveal this part of you. Take the time to let him get to know you first. And, conversely, get to know him. After the entrée, you may decide that you don't want this wally knowing all your intimate details. But if he is someone you think you could get close to, just remember to keep whatever you tell him in perspective. Yes, your cancer was a major life hurdle. But it wasn't your whole life and it shouldn't become a 400-pound gorilla sitting at the table with you.

If it's more comfortable for you, you can even wait until the very last moment to share your news. If you are confident with your body and you feel he is with you for *you*, there is nothing wrong with going upstairs to the bedroom, beginning foreplay, and then, as you start to undress, casually saying, "Oh, by the way, I had breast cancer a while back, so my breasts are awesome." Do you think he will want to stop? No way. On the other hand, if you approach the topic by say-ing, "I am really self conscious, I had breast cancer, and I hate how I look," you won't exactly send him reeling. You will also be sending the signal that you are still living in Cancerland and are, therefore, not yet ready to move on with your life.

Dating has never been easy. Dating after breast cancer is even harder. Like everything else in this journey, though, it will have its fits and starts, but it will smooth out as you find your groove. Fur-thermore, believe it or not, some men actually find that a woman who has been through so much and is back standing tall, living her life as a true survivor, is just the kind of woman they want! And you know what? They couldn't be more right.

MOTHERHOOD . . . OR NOT

Another harsh reality single survivors face is that if they didn't have children before their diagnosis, they may lose the dream of becoming a mom naturally post-diagnosis. Chemo can put you into premature menopause, and if it doesn't, your doctor may do so surgically or chemically. Hormone-sensitive cancers require the removal or block-ing of the hormones required to become pregnant and sustain a preg-nancy. One drug that is often prescribed to block these hormones is Tamoxifen, which you will most likely need to be on for at least five years. Where will you be in five years? Will you be menopausal then? Is it possible that you won't be able to have a baby? This is one of the hardest things for single survivors to accept. Yet, hardly anyone ever hears about this heartbreak, let alone discusses it candidly.

Deciding what you will do about motherhood is a major dilemma; maybe one of the biggest you will ever face. If you stop your post-therapy treatment and get pregnant, you will fill your body with an explosion of hormones—the same hormones that fed your cancer. Even if you had triple-negative disease, meaning your cancer was not fed by hormones, it is just as dangerous for you to get pregnant. It is not unheard of for a triple-negative woman to get a recurrence of estrogen-sensitive breast cancer. So how do you decide? Do you take the chance and risk recurrence for a baby? And if you do get a recurrence, how will it affect your baby growing up? Will you be there?

If you decide you want to at least have the option of becoming a mother naturally, you can harvest your eggs before your chemotherapy begins. This way they are preserved, and someday in the future you can get in vitro fertilization and have your baby. If you are financially and emotionally able, you also have the option of having a surrogate carry the baby for you if you harvest your eggs. The problem, however, is that no one tells you about this in the beginning when it's still an option.

ADOPTION

If it's too late to harvest your eggs, all is not lost. You can choose to adopt. Adoption gives you a second chance at fulfilling your mommy dreams, and your adopted child will be as much your own as a natural child would be. *If* you can get a baby, that is.

Unfortunately, the normal route to adoption—the public route—discriminates against women who have had breast cancer. Apparently, we are a bad risk. So "bad" that babies who need homes are denied loving ones simply because the adoption agencies erroneously feel that we will be dead soon. Last time I checked, we *survived* an awful disease and we're alive. What do they know?

Fortunately, there are ways around this false stereotype. For instance, you can privately adopt a baby if you have the money to do so. Since you are paying for the birth mother's prenatal living expenses and medical costs, and since she knows you are a survivor and still agrees to let you adopt her child, your chances at getting a baby are much better. A private adoption requires an attorney who specializes in this type of family law. What will happen is that a pregnant mom will make an arrangement with you, through the attorney, to give you her baby when it is born. You will have to pay legal fees, as well as cover the cost of the mom's living and medical expenses while she carries the baby. The biggest downside to this option is that there is a chance she could change her mind at the last moment, and there is nothing you can do about it. This is something you definitely need to be aware of when going into private adoption, so be sure to ask your attorney for all of the details.

Another alternative option is to do an overseas adoption, which as you may know, is a choice that is gaining in popularity. There are many orphans from war-torn and impoverished regions around the world who are looking for loving homes. This would be an international, private adoption. The costs vary depending on the country, so do your research. You should also know that the waiting time can be extremely long, the paperwork is quite extensive, and you will have to deal with foreign laws and governments. But you will get a baby. The baby may be a toddler, but it will be yours.

Now, there is no guarantee with any of this. But in order to adopt a baby you have to know all of your options. While the rules of public adoption may not accept you as a suitable parent since you're a cancer survivor, a pregnant woman who wants to give up her baby for adoption may not think twice about survival rates if she thinks you'll give her baby a loving home. If you adopt overseas you will have to cut through a lot of red tape, but you will be taking a baby out of a horrid situation and giving it a new life full of love and peace.

Finally, if you don't have the kind of money that a private or overseas adoption demands, there is another way. There are millions of foster children who need loving homes. They may be older and the arrangement may not be permanent, which is hard to fathom, but there is a good chance you could eventually adopt the child. At the very least, you will be providing love and happiness for a child who desperately needs it, and you will have the experience of being a parent. Check the laws in your state to educate yourself if you are interested in this option.

Losing the dream of natural motherhood is a devastatingly deep loss. It is one that must be acknowledged and mourned. If this is something you are facing, you undoubtedly feel a myriad of emotions, including guilt. And you have probably thought back to that old boyfriend you could have married but didn't—thinking if you had stayed together you would have a baby now. Don't dwell in the past, though, because nothing you do can change it. You left him for a reason. And it was the right reason for you. All you can do is make the best future possible for yourself. Instead of hanging your head and giving up, adjust your mindset, dream new dreams, and make new plans.

MAKE A NEW PLAN

Cancer and all that came with it was not in your plan. So what? Make a new plan. Do what you can now to make the best of it. You can even reinvent who you are and who you want to become. The first step in doing this is being kind to yourself. We want everyone else to be gentle and understanding with us, so why can't we demand the same from ourselves?

Take action to make yourself look and feel better. Your body, your image, your life-view, and your future are all new. Nothing is set in stone. If you don't like your reconstruction, get it revised or get a different one. If your lumpectomy scars and divots make you uncomfortable, get them corrected. If, after second thought, you decide that maybe you will give reconstruction a try and not live without breasts, research which doctors in your area do the best work.

It is perfectly understandable to be so worn out from everything you have been through to never want another procedure again, but if it will make a difference in the quality of your life and how you view yourself, suck it up and go for it. Similarly, if your face has seen happier days, look at page 45 and consider a few minor changes that can make a big difference in how you look and feel about yourself. Focus on your diet and exercise, and start rebuilding a stronger, healthier, less-likely-to-recur, you.

The point of all of this is that when you are actively working toward looking the best you can, you start to reclaim control over your life. With that control, you start to feel empowered. And with that empowerment, comes a sense of a newfound sexuality.

10

$\int$ex and the Single Survivor

The past year or so seems like a blurry dream, doesn't it? You know it's not because if you pinch yourself you can feel it, but you're still unsure about how you're supposed to feel about the person looking back at you in the mirror. Who is she and how can you feel connected to her again? If you want to find love, you have to reconcile with the new you and appreciate all you have been through and overcome. Once you love the person you see, others will start to, too.

Think of your body as a mighty ship. It has carried you through some stormy waters, and it has weathered the blustering wind and the blazing sun. At times you became sea sick, but you recovered and found your way back to safe harbor—to home. Looking at her hull in dry dock, the old girl shows some wear with a barnacled bottom, peeling paint, and a tear in the main sail. But she is sea worthy and you know that should she ever need to navigate rough seas again, she could do it.

After all your ship has done for you, it's time for you to take care of her. Scrape the bottom. Shine up the brass. Sew the main sail, or better yet, get her a new one. Your ship may not be the newest model in port, but it is a classic with great lines. She was built for joyful days in the open water. She is a pleasure craft, so don't store her in a ship-yard someplace—get her back out there.

FIND A FELLOW TRAVELER

To take this metaphor one step further, ask yourself who you want taking this ship out for a sail. Do you want to trust her to a day tripper who will not navigate her well, maybe tangle her lines, or put her in too close to the shallow waters near the rocks? How about a careless sailor who wears the wrong shoes and doesn't respect her newly painted deck? Or, would you rather trust her to an experienced captain who respects her lines, appreciates her sea-worthiness, wears Topsiders because he respects her body and doesnt want to scratch her in any way, enjoys taking her out to great depths, and deftly steers her with the wind?

Don't waste your time with day-tripper men. Why be dragged into the shallow waters of one night stands or flings? It's great that you have the urge to be out in the bay, but don't waste that urge on a man who does not appreciate you. Don't settle because you think he is the best you can do with your altered, "less-womanly" body. You are not any less of a woman! You had an illness and you did what was necessary to rid yourself of it. So, you have some scars. Real men don't see scars, but day trippers do. They act like they are doing you a favor or a service by being with you. Did you do months of chemo and radiation and have umpteen surgeries to be treated this way? Is this what you were fighting for? No way.

You fought for your life and you have it now, so make it the best life ever. That means never settling because you are feeling insecure or not complete as a woman. Resist the easy way out. Don't throw in the towel and say, "The heck with it. I'll just be alone the rest of my life." That is not living and you know it.

Some things are worth waiting for. A real man is one of those things. A real man who sees the beauty in you—a beauty that is enhanced by all that you have endured. William Butler Yeats beautifully described the kind of man worth waiting for in his poem "When You are Old":

> *"How many loved your moments of glad grace;*
> *And loved your beauty with love false or true;*

But one man loved the pilgrim soul in you,
And loved the sorrows of your changing face."

Find a fellow traveler. Find a man who loves the changes in you because they make you so much more of a woman. Perfect, unscathed women are a dime a dozen. Pilgrim souls—you—are rare and precious.

EMBRACE YOUR PILGRIM SOUL

What exactly is your pilgrim soul? Your pilgrim soul is what carried you through your journey and beyond. You may have had other people around you that were supporting you, but no one else could take your journey for you. You couldn't take a pass. You couldn't hire someone else to endure what you did. Only you know what it took. Only you know the pieces of your heart that were touched every time you were handled and prodded by the legions of experts at work making you well again.

There is a loneliness there . . . and a fear. A fear that is deep and real. A fear that haunts you like a looming cloud just beyond the horizon. You wonder whether there is another storm coming; whether you will be spared. Fortunately, your pilgrim soul is there to keep you looking forward—to keep your back to what may be looming ahead. In short, it helps you cope. You become paralyzed if you stay in the land of "what if's." Your pilgrim soul will keep you moving by looking to the land of "what will be's"—to the thousands of possibilities that lay ahead. And those possibilities include love.

It takes a very special man to recognize what you have been through. He may never completely understand it unless he, himself, has been touched by cancer or a life-threatening disease. But know that a man who "gets you" is out there. There is a man who will see you for what you are: Perfection that has been challenged, overcome, and regained. As a result, you will be even more beautiful in his eyes. It won't matter one whit what your reconstruction looks like. For him, it will go so much deeper. A woman who can fight like you have and can then stand up to the world again and say, "Here I am! I am back, I am strong, and I am ready to live!" is probably the most desirable of all women in the world. You are more than a woman now. And it takes more of a man to appreciate all that is you.

Beautiful, single sisters, pay attention to the day-tripper warning. One wrong night with a heartless man can set you back months. You have to protect your heart. You are vulnerable now, more so than you ever have been. Once you get over that first time with someone new, with your new body, you will be fine. But that is all the more reason to make that first man, the right man. There is a world of men out there and it is imperative to have your eyes open. It will be so easy to believe anything now, but therein lies the danger. Always keep in your mind these questions:

- Does he see me for who I am?

- Can he appreciate my pilgrim soul?

- Is he someone with whom I want to share this beautiful body that I fought so hard to save?

- Will he honor me?

- Does he want me for me, or as a conquest?

- Do I really want him?

When you find the right man for you, you will have the opportunity to rewrite your own life story. If your pre-breast cancer self didn't make the best of choices, if she did things you cringe at now, if she didn't make things special enough, then now is the time to welcome the new, exciting, enticing you into your fresh life story.

HAVING SEX FOR THE SAKE OF HAVING SEX

You haven't had sex in at least a year, because you were too busy refereeing a steel cage match between your DNA and cancer. You have been "keeping it busy," but you want to have *sex*; you want to feel a man in your arms again. You also want to get it over with—to see if your body still works like it used to. And finally, you are simultaneously curious and terrified to see your new body through the eyes of a lover.

If this sounds like you and you are itching to have sex for the sake of having sex, think about your options. Many women have an old boyfriend in the back of their closet someplace. Someone who, if you call him up, will come over. If you don't have that, you can always say yes to the guy at the gym or coffeeshop who keeps flirting with you. Regardless, you have no intention of making this a long term relationship. Basically, this is a booty call.

If you truly just want to see how the plumbing is working, go for it. However—and I'm sure you knew there would be a however—prepare yourself for the worst, just in case. After all, even if you have no feelings for someone, you are about to expose the most vulnerable parts of your new body to him. You are going to see whether or not your post-treatment body works with someone who doesn't give a crap about it, and the reality is that you may get hurt.

Since this is a booty call, he won't be sensitive to your needs. He won't think about how his facial expression as you take off your top will impact you. He may not be gentle, he may not take the time to get you fully ready for sex, and it may hurt. Know this going in. Meaningless sex is just that. Lovemaking is a whole different matter. If you're eager to have sex, though, and can handle the situation, go for it.

BE CONFIDENT IN YOURSELF

If you think you're sexy—if you really believe it—you will transfer that vibe to all who come into contact with you. A confident, bright-eyed woman who walks tall exudes sex appeal. Conversely, a woman who shlubs around in sweats and never makes eye contact, well, she does not exude anything positive.

Get yourself to a place where you honestly think, "Hot damn, I look great. I had cancer and look how awesome I am doing now." Then, when you are out in the world others will think the same way if you really believe in yourself. Do your best to fake it until you are honestly there. If you have to force yourself out of your shell, do it. Soon you will see that women who never had breast cancer don't have anything on you. You really are the superhero among your friends and family!

When the new, confident you steps out, don't be surprised if some small-minded, jealous types are a bit put out because you "shouldn't" look this great. Remember, they are also wondering why you are not hiding in your garden apartment. Ignore them and rock on. Show up back on the scene as a healthy, fantastic-looking survivor. Go ahead and shake up your skeptics! Females and males alike will all be a little taken aback by this new warrior angel.

SEPARATING THE MEN FROM THE BOYS

Unfortunately, the members of the male gender don't come labeled. We females have to find out the hard way if we are with a boy or a man. Fortunately, they do send out some signals. The trick is to know what they are so we can recognize them.

One tip is that all males fear inadequacy. They are afraid they are not good in bed, are not well-endowed, and can't please a woman. That doubt is in every boy and man. The difference lies in how they deal with it. Real men don't boast about their prowess in order compensate. But boys, on the other hand, tend to brag incessantly about how good and big they are. Most of the time, the more they talk the worse they are. The following lists lay out a few more signals to help you distinguish between boys and men.

Men

- Real men don't boast about what great lovers they are; they don't have to.

- Real men don't discuss their penises with ladies. They don't have to.

- Real men ask how you are feeling and genuinely want to know the answer.

- Real men think that what you went through is admirable and astonishing.

- Real men think that your experiences make you more desirable.

- Real men treat you like a precious jewel.

- Real men court you until you feel completely comfortable with them.

- Real men make love.

- Real men take their time and tell you that you are beautiful.

- Real men make sure you are satisfied.

Boys

- Boys tell you about how they've brought all the women in their past to multiple orgasms.

- Boys tell you that they are huge and that you should prepare for their girth.

- Boys want to make sure you know how they are feeling.

- Boys think what you went through is okay, as long as it doesn't affect their ability to get off.

- Boys think your experiences make you a charity case.

- Boys act like they are doing you favor by being with you.

- Boys want to jump in the sack right away. They don't want to waste time with dinner or conversation.

- Boys screw you.

- Boys want you to tell them how hot they are.

- Boys only worry about themselves. If you aren't satisfied it's your problem, not theirs.

Respect yourself and demand attention from the kind of men who can not only handle the strong, warrior angel that you are now, but who revel in it. You may not believe this, but there are men who think that someone who has done all that you have done and who has come out swinging, is more desirable than any other woman out there. These men are confident, aware, smart, and savvy. They think they have seen every type of woman—until you come along, proud and strong. Do not settle for any man who is less than this, and believe me, you will not find them among the boys of the world. The self-involved, shallow, narrow-minded Neanderthals just don't get it, and they definitely won't get you.

PERSONAL STORY: JENNY'S BOY STORY

Jenny had an experience with a boy that she had been friends with for years. Things got heated between them and they were almost ready to move to the next level. But then, she found out she had breast cancer and needed a bilateral mastectomy. Two years later, Jenny and the boy reconnected. It was the first time she had been with anyone since her surgery.

Jenny was understandably terrified. She was very open with him and told him that she had not been with anyone in years. She also told him that she had reconstructed breasts, and that she was terribly unsure about them because she had not yet seen them through a man's eyes. Over the years he had often regaled her with tales of his sexual prowess. She had heard story after story of women left weak with delight over the multiple orgasms he was able to give them. He had also bragged about his size and warned her that most women swooned at the very sight of him. So now, when she was about to be the object of his desire, he told her that he would bring her back to her sexual self, and that she would be as fulfilled as any woman could ever hope to be.

Excited, Jenny and the boy decided to go to a little Inn for the weekend. After a delicious meal, they went up to their room. Jenny was petrified. How she had managed to swallow any of her dinner was a miracle to her.

Eventually, the moment of truth came. Sitting on top of him, Jenny slowly removed her lacey bra. She took a deep breath and exposed her breasts to someone who was not a doctor for the first time since her surgeries. Unfortunately, his reaction crushed her. He blankly stared and said nothing. He didn't say she was beautiful and he didn't reassure her that she was not the freak she was afraid she was. In fact, he looked a bit repulsed. It was hard for Jenny to move forward, but she swallowed her mortification and they continued.

It was now his turn. It was time for his big reveal. To this day, Jenny is still wondering why she didn't swoon like the other women he told her about had. But even though he didn't make her go weak in the knees, she told him he looked great. She treated him the way he should have treated her, by stroking his ego . . . among other things. Then, he started his technique—his "internationally famous" technique. Is it any surprise to learn he over-promised? This boy, who said he had never left a woman's bed without her being satisfied multiple times in a row, finished for himself and then rolled over and went to sleep.

Jenny tortured herself the whole night. Lying there, she convinced herself that she was permanently disfigured and that no man would ever want her again. Then, as if the previous night hadn't been enough, over breakfast he told her that she "needed to work on her orgasm." Jenny felt like a spotlight was on her. It was, according to him, her fault that she did not climax the night before.

The second night at the Inn, Jenny had to initiate the sex. She had never had to do that before. Before cancer, men always wanted her and made sure she knew it. The sex the second time around was no better. He reached climax and rolled over and went to sleep. On the third night, neither of them even attempted sex even though it was their last night together. She slept on her side of the bed and he slept on his. At that moment, Jenny decided that there would not be another night with this boy. He had shattered her ego for the last time.

For a couple of weeks after that weekend, Jenny, like most women, blamed herself, her reconstruction, and her cancer. She was convinced she would never know love or wonderful sex again. It took space and time to let the dust settle before she saw the entire encounter in perspective. She took off her rose-colored glasses and saw what he looked like. He wasn't bad looking, but he wasn't a god. Here she was worried about her body, when his was not anything to boast about. And on top of that, he was not a good lover. A good lover cares about his partner's needs as well as his own. Ultimately, she realized that he was not a nice person, either. He had treated her poorly and she knew she deserved better.

Jenny sat back and smiled. She was worried about what her implants looked like? It wasn't her, it was *him*. He was the wrong guy. What's more, he was a fool. If he was as smart and as in touch with women as he claimed to be, he would have known that all he had to do was tell her she was beautiful and look at her with desire. If he had done that, she would have become more aroused and felt sexy, and the passion would have been intense. But, because he was so inept at personal interaction and had no thoughts of anyone other than himself, he just laid there like a king thinking he was doing her a favor.

It was then that Jenny decided she would no longer waste her time with boys. She was going to find a man. A real man.

PERSONAL STORY: ANNIE'S MAN STORY

Annie lived in the gate house on a large estate in Virginia's horse country, where there are still estates and manor houses to be found. Her house was nestled in the woods not far from the manor house, and she took care of things for the owners when they traveled, which was often.

Kevin worked for the owners of the horse farm. He had to come out there quite often, so she had known him for years. He saw her when she was in chemo—when she looked awful. But she figured since she was home, it didn't matter to her what she looked like. She inevitably ran into him on the estate when she was not looking her best, usually dressed in her sweatpants, her face bloated from the steroids, and what was left of her hair in a ratty pony tail—she had a lumpectomy and did the type of chemo that did not make her lose all of her hair, only part of it. But regardless, Kevin was always warm and smiling, and she thought he was lovely and sweet. They would say hello, chat a bit, and then she would return to the safety of the gate house that had become her bunker in her war against cancer.

When her treatments were finally over, Annie took a long time to heal. She had a long year of surgeries and treatments, and the after-effects lingered. She was also very depressed without even realizing it. She didn't see herself as a woman anymore. She literally saw herself as a permanent cancer patient, who might as well be wearing a hospital gown and dragging around an IV pole.

Even so, she realized that Kevin was as handsome a man as she had ever known. He had piercing blue eyes and perfect features. His smile could make her melt. He was funny and smart, and they laughed at each other's jokes. She felt a strong attraction to him and the feeling was mutual. In fact, the air crackled with electricity when they were together. But he was married with kids, and Annie was not about to go there. She would never go out with a married man, nor would she even entertain a fantasy about it. She knew that affairs with married men may be heaven in the beginning, but that they quickly turned to hell on earth.

Annie finished all her treatments in July and spent the rest of the summer healing on the outside, but simply existing on the inside. The summer turned to fall and she felt the new season better suited her mood. Then, winter set in and Annie's days bled into one another with no real change. She saw Kevin off and on at the main house when she had to let him in so he could work in the office while the owners traveled. The attraction they had for each other was still strong. One day, he actually verbalized how attracted he was to her by saying that if he wasn't married, he would want to be with her. Annie melted. It was a little drop of water on the desert that was her low self-esteem and self-imposed exile from the rest of the human race. But she quickly dismissed it as him just being kind to the nice girl with cancer.

Time continued to pass uneventfully until one late afternoon in April when the phone rang. It was the estate owner, who was in Europe at the time, saying he needed Annie to contact Kevin so that he could take care of a problem at the house. When she finally reached Kevin, he said he could be over first thing in the morning. And then it happened. He said, "Would you like to have dinner with me tonight?"

Annie was taken aback. She replied, "You are married." He said, "Not anymore I'm not." According to Kevin, he and his wife had been separated for months. He was living at a friend's house and had not been able to think of anyone but Annie. She took a deep breath and said yes.

Annie opened her closet door. There was nothing but drab, bleak clothing that permanent cancer patients wear in there. She had once been cute with great style. But since she had become the equivalent of the living dead, her wardrobe had begun to reflect it. She eventually found a couple of items to try on, but then started to feel nervous about the whole concept. She thought maybe she should cancel. After all, it would be so much easier to just stay home, watch TV, and forget the whole thing. Then she remembered his smile . . . and those eyes . . .

As she dressed, she looked at her scars. She had a lumpectomy scar and a divot where the tissue was removed. Her left breast was a darker color than her right one because of the radiation, which also caused it to sit a little higher. How could she ever let a man see her like this? How could she possibly even entertain the thought of a date—a date with a man so handsome he could have any woman he wanted? Getting dressed and leaving her house was one of the hardest things she had ever done. She was very nervous and in completely unfamiliar waters. But she did it.

When she arrived at the restaurant, she stood at the bar and noticed that there was an incredibly handsome man waving and smiling in her direction. Out of curiosity, she turned around to see who he was waving to. It was then that she realized the man was Kevin, and that he was waving at her. A man that gorgeous was waving to Annie? Was this real? She remembered her pre-cancer looks and how she was considered pretty. But now . . . now she didn't consider herself anything. Did Kevin see something in her that she did not?

She joined him and almost immediately, old feelings that she thought were long dead came bubbling to the surface. She was smiling and laughing again, and yes, even flirting back at him! It had been such a long time since she had done any of those things, that it all seemed new. There was a band playing in the restaurant, so they ate dinner and enjoyed the music. When dinner was over, Annie started to lose her nerve. The night was going *too* well and their attraction was stronger than ever. She turned to Kevin and said it was late so she should be getting home. In response, he teased her and said, "Oh, that's right. You have to get up early to let me into the Manor house tomorrow morning." It was true, that was her only plan for the day and he knew it. But things were heating up quickly and Annie didn't know where to go with her feelings for him.

When he took her hand, she could scarcely breathe. He then leaned in and kissed her—the first kiss Annie had in years. It was the kind of kiss that makes the rest of the world disappear. They were no longer in a restaurant. They were the only two people left on earth. Annie eventually regained consciousness and stood up to leave. Her heart was racing. What was happening? Was this blood that was flowing in her veins again? She said goodnight to Kevin and left.

When she got to her car, she noticed the moon. It was full and bright, and she could smell spring in the air. It was an unusually warm night for April. She had left the gate house windows open, so the intoxicating night air was now inside. She removed her clothes, drew a bath in her deep, luxurious tub with claw feet, and thought about his kiss. She stepped into the fragrant waters and let her mind wander until it was interrupted by the phone. It was him.

"I can't stop thinking about you," he said.

"Where are you?" Annie asked.

"I'm nearby in my car."

Annie didn't respond. She couldn't. She didn't know what to say to him. Finally, she said, "I will unlock the back door of the main house so you can let yourself in tomorrow morning. That way, you can come as early as you want without having to wait for me." She could hear him smiling, but he didn't say anything more. They hung up.

Annie leaned her head back again and inhaled the lavender-scented bath oil. But then she smelled something else—a cigarette. Cigarette smoke was weaving its way up into the window of the bathroom. She heard leaves rustling and the phone rang again.

"Where are you?" she asked him.

"I'm close by." Kevin said.

"Are you on the property?"

"Yes."

Annie jumped out of the tub and wrapped a towel around herself until she found her robe. With the phone still up to her ear, she walked into the bedroom and smelled the smoke coming in that window, too. She looked out into the driveway and saw his car. He then said into the phone, "Why don't you come downstairs? It's beautiful out tonight."

"What are you doing here?" she asked.

He said, "I forgot to kiss you goodnight."

And without so much as a second thought, she did it. Wearing just her robe with the hair on the back of her neck still wet with bath water, Annie walked out of the gate house. She walked out of the place that had been her shelter during her battle against breast cancer. She was leaving it behind. She was also leaving behind that permanent cancer patient. She walked out into the April night a woman again—a desirable, living woman. And she was embraced by the arms of one of the most beautiful men she had ever laid her eyes on.

When they made love, he opened her robe and exposed her breasts. She panicked and thought the earth would surely stop once he saw her ugly scars. Thankfully, only her heart did temporarily. He leaned over and kissed each scar lovingly, as if it was the most beautiful thing he had ever seen. A wave of relief flooded Annie. And so, too, did her desire. She thought that had died long ago, but here it was as strong as ever.

In fact, she discovered that she had become a more sensual lover than she had ever been. She savored every one of his touches and took her time exploring his body. There was no pain when they made love, just pleasure. Annie was reborn that night. She was a cancer survivor. And she had been made love to by a man who found her beautiful inside and out, and each of her scars made her only more lovely to him.

RULES OF THE DATING ROAD

In order to find the right person you have to keep both your heart and your eyes open. There aren't too many Knights in shining armor riding around on horseback anymore, but there are still plenty of good men—sweet and loving men—who are looking for their special woman as much as you are looking for your special man. Although there are no secrets to finding "The One," there are some rules you can follow that will help.

To Thine Own Self Be True

Do you want to find someone who is true to himself, self-confident, open, and sees life full of possibilities? If your answer is yes, you must first become that yourself. When you are comfortable in your own skin, it shows. Don't waste your time pretending to be someone else in order to win over someone you find attractive. You can't keep up a facade, nor should you want to! Let the real you show. You will be far more relaxed, and your date will have a better time learning about you. He will feel comfortable because you are comfortable.

Don't Play Mind Reader

Why we do this to ourselves is a mystery, but we really must stop. Don't try to read into what your date is saying or how he is acting. Don't presume he is turned off by you because you are a cancer survivor. However, with that being said, if all you do on the first date is talk in detail about how much chemo made you hurl, then maybe he really will be turned off. Chill out. If the topic of your cancer comes up, he may not know exactly what to say, but that doesn't mean he doesn't want to be there with you. Let things happen naturally. See how they unfold. Take the night off from being a detective and just *be*.

Chemistry is Overrated

You may not feel that "click" when you first meet your date. Maybe he's wearing sandals with socks. Or maybe you see a tattoo of a duck with the caption "Mr. Natural" on his arm that makes you want to escape out the back door of the restaurant. Don't leave. Give him a chance. Ask him about "Mr. Natural." There may be a great story behind it! Perhaps he got it when he was sixteen and has regretted it ever since. As far as the sandals with socks, well, there really is no excuse for that. But if it works out, you can encourage him to change his wardrobe. Open your heart and your mind. He may be a diamond in the rough, so give him at least two dates before you rule him out.

Be Realistic about "The One"

Alright, is this a myth or does he exist? One thing is for certain—you will never find out if you don't put yourself out there. He won't come to you while you are hanging out at home watching *Top Chef*. Get dressed and leave your house so you can meet him! There are many men that could become "The One," and it's important to be realistic. Your dream man may be a combination of several men from your life experience, which is undoubtedly a lot for a guy to live up to. So, when you're evaluating a new man, instead ask yourself if he has *most* of the qualities of your dream man. Winnow your list down a bit and try not to be overly judgmental. That being said, don't ever settle or lower your expectations too far. Trust yourself. Look into his heart. Look into *your* heart. And finally, keep these words from the dad in the movie *Juno* in mind: "Look, in my opinion, the best thing you can do is find a person who loves you for exactly what you are. Good mood, bad mood, ugly, pretty, handsome, what have you, the right person is still going to think the sun shines out your ass. That's the kind of person that's worth sticking with."

Shut Up

If you want a man to think you are the most fascinating woman in the world, then shut up. Let him talk about himself all night. When you say goodnight, he will think you are positively the most interesting woman he has ever met. You will also learn a lot. *Now* is the time to ask the questions you don't dare ask when the relationship starts to get more serious. Questions like, "Why did you break up with your last girlfriend?" "What did she look like?" "Did you cheat on her or did she cheat on you?" Pay attention. What you learn will help you understand him better, which in turn will help you figure out how to approach the subject of your own past with more knowledge of your audience.

Laughter is an Aphrodisiac

Having a good laugh, letting go, being silly, and cracking one another up brings out the kid in all of us. It makes us feel good, brings us closer together, and can eventually turn into some amazing love making. See the humor in everything. Life, and love, will be so much easier if you do.

Tell Him He Looks Good

Do you like what you see? Tell him! Make sure you are sincere, of course. If you like the way he looks in his jeans, tell him. If his hair looks nice, tell him. Men are just like us. They like to hear nice things about themselves. Remember this: Be wary of a man who never has anything nice to say about you. If you are wearing a beautiful dress and make a great entrance and he can't utter even a measly "wow," put him on your watch list. He may be very self-involved.

Keep Your Own Life Blossoming

Do not stop your life to become part of his—particularly if you are just in the beginning stages of your relationship. Don't phone, email, or text him incessantly. Be a little mysterious. This is also a good way to see how long it takes him to contact you. If you are contacting him all the time you can't judge that, now can you?

The Cure for Men is More Men

If he is a jerk . . . if he lets you down . . . if he doesn't say one nice thing about you . . . if he acts like he can't handle you because you had an illness . . . if he acts like he did you a favor because he was nice to the cancer patient . . . dump him! Disappear off of his radar. Then get back out into the dating world immediately. Join a new club, go out to a bar, sign up on a dating site—just do something. Start thinking about the possibilities of other men as soon as possible so you can forget that jerk.

Don't Go Deaf, Dumb, or Blind

You are really happy to have found someone who thinks you're beautiful and sexy, likes to sail, watches the same TV shows as you, and laughs at your jokes. Could this be love? Could you have truly conquered cancer and moved on with living? Maybe! But don't turn a blind eye to his bad traits—and yes, everyone has bad traits. Does he drink too much? You can't change that or get him to stop. Does he flirt with waitresses in front of you, look at other women, and even have a coterie of female pals online? He won't stop that and you can't change it. Does he spend money foolishly or act irresponsibly? You can't change that or make him clean up his act.

You can only change two things about a man: His clothes and his hair. The rest is never going to change. He may put on a show for a couple of months, but he will always revert back to his old habits. Don't be so desperate that you will be willing to marry a man who is an alcoholic, drug abuser, flirt, or spendthrift. Walk away. You don't need any more problems, do you?

Safety First

Must we really deal with this? Um, let's see. You finished chemo to rid yourself of cancer, you are taking hormonal medicine to protect yourself from cancer, but you don't insist on a condom? That is just plain and simply crazy. The last thing you need is another item on your medical history. Buy a box of condoms yourself and always make sure you have them on hand. Get the lubricated variety. Get two sizes—regular and large. Hey, you never know!

ONLINE DATING

If you live in an area that feels more like Noah's Ark than the set of *The Dating Game,* you may need to bring in outside help and work a little harder to find dates. There are many horror stories about online dating sites, but there are also many success stories. Be cautious and do your research, but keep an an open mind.

It's safe to say that the majority of men on Internet dating sites are window shopping. They're looking to see who is available, and over time, they build up a group of female friends with whom they chat. The problem is that this can go on for years. If you find yourself bantering back and forth endlessly with someone who never suggests actually meeting up with you, move on. Similarly, stay away if someone seems over-eager and sends you a note that says something like, "I like your picture. Let's have a cocktail. Send me your phone number *now.*"

If, however, you find someone who seems reasonably normal, ask him for his full name. If he gives it to you, Google him to find out who he is. You may find information that makes you even more excited about him, but, on the other hand, you may see a lovely picture of him with his wife and fourteen kids—because online dating isn't cheating, right? If he only gives you his email address, not his full name, you can still put that into a Google search and see what comes up. If you see that same email on questionable message forums, you have your answer. Google is great.

In addition to being aware of who you are talking to, you also need to be aware of what type of dating site you are on. For example, if you want sex and nothing else, there are dating websites—usually found in the back of magazines or advertised on late-night television—specifically designed for booty calls that will fill that need. On these websites, someone simply goes online and announces that he or she wants to get laid. Then, if someone else in the area wants to get laid, too, and likes how the other person looks, it is a done deal.

There are also more traditional and conservative dating websites. Match.com is probably the most well-known. Everyone and their cousin Seymour, literally, can join it for free and just lurk. However, you can only communicate with other members if you pay the membership fee, which is actually a good way to determine whether or not someone is serious about finding a partner or not. You will know you have someone serious if he has a lot of information and photos posted.

eHarmony is another traditional dating website. It essentially makes you take the equivalent of an SAT test before it sends you matches, and it is also the most expensive. However, the costly fee means that the members are serious romance seekers—perhaps that is why eHarmony is also the most successful. As with Match, if a man has little to no information or photos posted, don't even bother. Instead, go for a man who is open, revealing, and appears genuine. After all, if he took the time to take the SAT test, fill out a complete profile, and paid the bucks to be there, he may be seriously looking for you. Even so, still make sure you Google him before you meet him for coffee—in a public place of course. *Always* meet in public. Never give out your personal information until you know the person you are giving it to is not going to be appearing on next Friday's edition of *America's Most Wanted.*

And finally, for Pete's sake, you do *not* have to tell some guy you are emailing with on an online dating site about your breast cancer. Remember, he could be anyone. You don't know who someone is until—or if—you meet him. After you have been out with someone a couple of times and have decided that you want to get to know him more and that you want him to get to know you more, you can tell him. There is no rush to reveal your medical history.

IT'S NOT EASY, BUT YOU CAN DO IT

From pilgrim souls to *America's Most Wanted* . . . no one ever said being single was simple. Sprinkle in a little cancer and you have yourself quite a complex maze to figure out. No matter what happens, though, honor yourself. Like Dorothy in the *Wizard of Oz*, you always have the ability to find your way home again. You also found the Lion's courage when you needed it the most to fight your cancer. You had the Scarecrow's brain when you needed to make all those decisions. And, even though your heart was broken when you were diagnosed, like the Tin Man, it is still beating strong.

Look within and love yourself for all you were, all you are, and all you can and will be. Then look around you. Find someone who can see who you really are. Find someone who, the more he sees, the more he wants to know you and be close to you.

You are confident and sexy, and you can take care of yourself. You are aware of what to look out for, as well as what to look for, in a man. Don't lock yourself up and throw away the key just because you had cancer. Your whole life is in front of you; go out and grab it.

11

$\mathcal{Y}$our Style

Feeling sexy and looking great is not a costume change out of a catalog; it is a lifestyle change. Getting in touch with your inner goddess means getting into the right frame of mind, taking care of your body and your future health, making yourself look as good as you can, learning how to express your feelings, and sharing your fears and desires with those you love. Feeling and looking your best should not be saved solely for special occassions. It should be part of your daily life—the whole new life that you have reclaimed. So, married or single, it's time to come together and get down to what we are wearing, how we are wearing it, and how we can set the stage for romance and the best sex of our lives.

WHAT TO WEAR

After you have worn paper examination capes, flimsy hospital gowns, and let's not forget those utterly charming blue surgical caps, you should truly appreciate how nice your clothes are. And there is no denying it: If you look good, you feel good. Pay attention to how you look, because it does, quite often, reflect how you feel. And you can change your whole attitude with just a simple change of clothes! If you know you took an extra five minutes in the morning to look your best, you'll have more confidence throughout the rest of the day.

Are You in Uniform?

There is a new "uniform" that many women of today wear every-where. It consists of a hoodie or oversized t-shirt on top, and either mom jeans or too-tight sweatpants with "cute" wording emblazoned cheek-to-cheek on bottom. When not sporting this fashion-don't, some women even leave the house wearing actual pajama bottoms—in public! Are you a member of the team that wears this uniform? If your answer is yes, then it is time to change your style. You already had your body changed for you by cancer; don't make matters worse. Make things better.

How? After you have put on some deliciously scented body lotion and your matching lingerie of the day, think twice before you reach for your ratty hoodie that has seen better days. Instead, take a good look in your closet. Is that the cashmere sweater that your mom gave you for your birthday back there? Why aren't you wearing it? What are you saving it for? Put it on!

If you have a nice skirt—something simple and straight—why not put that on, too? And then complete the look with some cute ankle boots, stylish knee-high boots, or some pretty, kitten-heeled pumps. Let's face it, ballet flats look great and stylish on women like Audrey Hepburn. But do you have a body like hers? If you don't, ballet flats can turn your lovely ankles into cankles—the not-so technical term for a calf that turns into a foot—thereby obliterating the graceful curve of an ankle. Boots that make you look like you're ready for a lunar walk aren't so attractive, either. Pay close attention to how you look in footwear. It can make or break your outfit, and make or break how slender or fat your legs look, too.

Okay, so you still need to be practical. You are not about to wear a skirt for day-to-day things and sometimes you really just need to wear jeans. That's fine. But do your homework. Do they come all the way up your torso, turning them into mom jeans? Do they make your butt look like a pancake? Or conversely, do the tiny pockets make your butt look like it belongs to Gigantor? Study your body type. Then, find the proper style of jeans to go with it. And always, always look at yourself in a three-way mirror before buying a new pair.

As a general frame of reference, lower-rise jeans will make your butt look smaller. But if your belly is big, don't wear a low-cut jean that it will hang over; a muffin-top isn't a good look on anyone. Boot cut jeans makes wide hips seem narrower, because they balance out your body. Additionally, the bigger the pocket, the smaller your butt will look. And if you don't want to call attention to your butt, don't wear jeans with sequins on the back pockets. There are jeans with built-in tummy control, but be careful with these as they skirt dangerously close to the mom-jean category. If the pair you try on would go perfectly with an appliquéd sweater with smiling pumpkins on it, they are mom jeans.

Another thing to take into consideration when buying jeans is the wash. Everyone looks better in a dark wash. Whoever thought up the bleaching out of jeans around the fattest part of a woman's butt had to be a man who didn't like women very much. You might as well have on a flashing neon sign that says, "Right here! This is where I store my fat! Did I highlight it enough for ya?"

The bottom line is this: Try on all the clothes in your closet and look in the mirror to see how they fit your body. Throw out or give to charity the clothes that don't do anything for you. If you can get an honest second opinion, definitely do. If you can't, set your camera on its timer and take a picture of yourself in each outfit. You can get a good idea of how things really look that way. If your clothes are showing wear, are frayed, have pills in the fabric, or simply don't flatter your body, throw them out or give them away if they are in good shape.

Everyday Lingerie

There is a lot of advice out there telling you to not worry about how you look when it comes time to be intimate with a man. People think all it takes is some lace here and there. Women are told to buy some sexy bras to feel more attractive when they retire to the bedroom with their partners. There's absolutely nothing wrong with that, but the question is, why are you only letting yourself feel more attractive when it is time to take your clothes off? Why are you only wearing your good stuff for your man?

You have scars now—both on the outside and on the inside. The inner scars are directly affected by your reaction to the outer scars. Yet, some women give up after breast cancer and simply throw on a pair of sweats or jeans and a baggy shirt, and schlep through their days looking like the ragged end of nowhere. If this sounds like your routine, is there any wonder why you don't feel attractive?

Since you have to live in a new body every day, why not make it special every day? Go out and get lingerie. Match your bras to your panties and never mix and match them again. The secret to this is to buy one amazing-style bra and a few pairs of matching panties. If you do this with a couple of different styles and colors, you will have the foundation of a great new collection of lingerie.

Once you have them, wear them *every day*. Yes, every single day. Then, instead of harboring the secret, inner-dread of your scars underneath your clothes, your focus will be on the delicate, lacy lingerie you are wearing. It will change your whole outlook. You will stand up taller and smile a little broader. You will feel sexy and attractive. And do you want to know the best part? You will be doing it for you, not for some man you are married to or who you may meet and eventually be intimate with.

The power of everyday lingerie can make you feel very beautiful and desirable again. Just think, while you are watching your child's soccer practice and looking at all the other moms with their never-been-sick bodies, instead of feeling less of a woman than they are, you can smile to yourself and think of how pretty the satin ribbons and pearl detail of your bra and panties look and feel on you. These women are probably wearing mismatched underwear! You know better.

Every day should be a special day, and that should be reflected in your garments—both the ones that are seen by the public and the ones that only you know you are wearing. Throw out the mindset that, "No one knows what I am wearing underneath, so who cares?" And replace it with, "Never leave the house without beautiful, matching, sexy lingerie, because life is too short for anything else!"

Bedroom Lingerie

While you are buying your hot new panties and bras, take a look at some of the nightgowns. Feel the satin and lace. Even cotton nightgowns can be delicate and pretty. Pick out and purchase a few of your favorites, and don't go to bed in an old t-shirt and mismatched pajama bottoms ever again.

Many women who choose not to reconstruct feel they have fewer options. However, even though they may not have "new" breasts, they still have plenty of things they can wear that will make them feel sexier. If you have chosen not to reconstruct, pick out your sexiest bra and wear it when you make love. It is said that Marilyn Monroe slept in a bra and Sarah Jessica Parker did all her love scenes in *Sex and the City* wearing a bra—there is nothing un-sexy about it! You may find, though, that it is totally unnecessary because your partner appreciates the real you more than you ever imagined. He doesn't need a bra or lingerie. He just needs you. He doesn't care about your breasts. You are more than your breasts to him. What a wonderful feeling that is!

If you had a single mastectomy, then you still have one breast. That means that you still have all the sensation and all the pleasures of touch on that side that you lost on the other with your mastectomy. So, while making love, make use of the one you still have! Make your sexy bra come off seductively on that side. It makes for a very alluring picture.

But no matter what kind of surgery you had or didn't have, take the time to pamper yourself and explore your sensual side. Take a bath before bed. Put on body lotion. Slip into a beautiful nightgown and dab on some of your favorite perfume. Do this whether you are with someone or all alone. It is all about how it makes you feel.

By taking care of yourself, treating yourself well, and indulging in simple things, you will start to feel better. You will also begin to feel more in tune with your body and by extension, you will feel sexier. When your confidence is high and you are feeling great, you are ready to open yourself up to the next step. Awaken your inner goddess. She is there and she is waiting for you to call on her. When you take care of yourself, she comes out.

If you are concerned about how your breasts—or lack of breasts—look, then don't make them the focal point. What about the rest of you? When getting ready to be with your lover, your inner goddess will help you if you listen to her. Make sure the skin on your legs is soft and stubble free. Moisturize. Take extra time on your hair. Play up your eyes. These are all things you can do to make you look your best and feel empowered. The focus is not just on your breasts anymore. It is on who you are as a whole. You are a goddess and you should let the world know it.

HOW TO TALK TO YOUR PARTNER ABOUT SEX

Lovemaking is a beautiful duet of bodies, minds, and feelings. You and your partner are in it together, so you should both feel comfortable discussing it with one another. And although you may not have had detailed conversations about sex before, now that you have extenuating circumstances with your "new" body, you need to. Bringing joy back to your life is the most healing and fulfilling gift you can give yourself. Always remember that you are worth it. You need to open up the dialogue with your lover. It is worth putting yourself out there and suggesting things that will make your lovemaking better.

Talk Sooner Rather than Later

Don't let the fear of your partner's reaction keep you from having discussions about sex. Your happiness is just as important as his. And if you are enjoying your lovemaking more, he will enjoy it more, too. Whatever you do, don't let things sit and fester. If you wait too long to mention something, you risk getting to the point of no return where you can no longer bring up what you really wanted to talk about. So, as things occur to you, or if certain things don't feel right, speak up right away. The same holds true for things you enjoy. If you like something he does, make sure he knows so he will do it again and again!

That being said, do be careful about how you say certain things, because he may interpret them differently than you intended. For instance, if you express a problem, he may feel guilty or inadequate. Therefore, it is important to reinforce that the bad guys are cancer and what you had to do to beat it, not him. In that context, he will be more open to suggestions.

Do you remember the show and tell exercise for overcoming breast numbness that we talked about earlier (page 84)? Now that you are more in sync with your body and know what works for you, instead of saying, "I hate when you do that," show him what you love. Say, "This sends me over the top," and then strategically place his hand wherever it feels good. This will get the point across without any confusion of what you are asking for, or any hurt feelings or bruised egos.

Positive reinforcement works wonders. When he is doing what you asked and it is amazing, tell him! Tell him what a great lover he is. Tell him you wish all women could have someone as caring and intuitive a lover as he is. This is especially important if you want him to remember to do it again! It all adds up to the most basic of instincts: Communication. Without it, we really are just flailing around. With it, we can move mountains, and each other.

Approach Certain Conversations with Care

Telling your partner about your toy chest may not be easy, particularly if you've never talked about such topics before. There is probably some level of embarrassment on your end and that is perfectly normal. You also have to be aware of his feelings. Tread lightly and slowly, and make sure you time the discussion correctly.

First, don't start the conversation when you are in the throes of passion. Pick a neutral time. One where neither of you will feel intimidated by the topic. Second, make sure he knows that it is not some inadequacy on his part that is causing you to bring toys into the mix. Your body is different now. You have to explain to him that in order to keep up your wonderful sex life, you have enhanced your personal belongings. Finally, take away the shame that may be associated with toys. You are not a degenerate. You are using what is necessary to maintain your sexual activity.

You can start by telling him you use a vibrator by yourself—a simple, level one vibrator with no bells or whistles. If you are really comfortable, show him how you use it. This will most likely be something he will want to see and will be more into it than you can ever imagine. When you have conquered that, and if he understands and shows interest, look online together at what else is available for you both to enjoy. This can be a very erotic activity. Furthermore, sitting at dinner knowing that the UPS guy dropped off a package from Babeland earlier in the day can be very exciting. It helps build the anticipation of what the two of you will be unwrapping and exploring later.

SLOW DOWN AND MAKE SEX LAST

Foreplay is of the utmost importance in helping you reconnect with your own body and the body of your lover. The longer you take, the better your lovemaking will be. Turn off the television, lock the doors, turn off the phones, and spend time on each other without any distractions. Transport yourself to another plane—one of pleasure and feeling good—and let go of all that may hold you back. There is an art to lovemaking and its canvas is foreplay. And without a good canvas, you cannot create a masterpiece.

The Art of Kissing

Nothing can ruin the potential for a great relationship like a bad kiss. Conversely, nothing can fool you into a bad relationship like a great kiss. This is because we are biologically wired to judge our potential mates by their kisses. No, really. There are scientists who study this phenomenon. It's called philematology. Basically, if we were to harken back to our cavewoman days, we would have a biological mechanism that would allow us to judge if we were with the right mate simply by swapping saliva. Today, a kiss tells us more about our chemistry with another person than anything else can.

If pheromones pull us in through scent, then kissing pulls us in through taste. Saliva contains hormones, so your mate can actually transfer testosterone to you through a long, slow, wet kiss that lasts three days, as Kevin Costner described in *Bull Durham*. Since we hormone-deprived women can use all the help we can get, and since testosterone has been shown to increase arousal, perhaps there really is something to this foreplay.

That being said, could this boost of testosterone also be given to the vagina naturally through oral sex? This is only a theory now, and it needs further study. However, many women have found that long sessions of oral sex before intercourse makes them more lubricated, aroused, and able to have pain-free penetration without any worries of atrophy. Therefore, doctors are formulating testosterone into a gel for women to use topically before sexual activity. What all this means is that now that you are a cancer survivor, your quickie days are over.

Long Live the Longie

You were a hot lover before cancer. You know you were. You took chances and probably had more than one quickie in an inappropriate spot. That is all fun and games, but is that the sex that was the most satisfying for you? Think back. What lovemaking sessions are seared in your brain? The quickie you had in the elevator even though you knew your boss was on the first floor waiting for the same elevator and would see you looking more than a little flushed? Okay, so maybe you will remember that one. . . . But seriously, think about it. Think about that time where you spent hours making love. It started with talking, then kissing and petting, and then the lovemaking that lasted and lasted. Those sessions are the ones that make romance novels and soap opera plots seem tame.

Now is the time to bring that passion back. Say goodbye to quickies. It is time to enter the world of longies. A longie involves talking, flirting, kissing, hugging, and caressing. A longie holds the promise of moonlight in a martini. You both know where the night is going, and the longer you wait for it to begin, the better it will be.

Make the night leading up to your longie an event, complete with fresh flowers, the right music, and a couple of candles. Spend an hour in the tub soaking in your favorite bath oil. Moisturize with a body lotion that matches your perfume. Make sure your hair is clean and soft. Spray some of your perfume onto your brush and pull it through your hair, but go easy applying perfume on your body. First, you don't want to smell like your Aunt Edna, and second, perfume tastes bad when licked.

Pick out some special lingerie from your new collection and slip it on. Have a drink. Play some music that means something to you to get you in the mood. Remember when you were in college or your early twenties and you thought you were the hottest thing on earth? Play some of the songs that got you in the mood back then. Never underestimate the power that Blondie and Led Zeppelin have to take you back in time. When your date arrives, tone the music down to jazz or something equally sensual and slow, so you can set and keep a pace for your impending longie.

Spend the night enjoying each other's company stress-free. You have already had the cancer talk. He knows you are a Warrior Princess. He knows your body has been enhanced by all it has endured, and similarly, he knows you need some lubrication so don't be shy about it. Set up a silver tray next to your bed with a selection of lubricants and put a rose on it. If you are really confident, share some of your toys with him.

Explore every inch of each other's bodies. If you want to keep your bra on, that is fine. Just make it an incredibly sexy bra. Use certain words that spark desire. "I want you" is one hot sentence. It projects power, lust, and the potential for great things to come. Leave Cancer Girl outside the door. She is not who you are anymore. She is not invited to your longie. And the deeper you delve into this essential part of your inner being, the farther away from you she will go.

The bottom line is this: Make sex last. Make it fun. Make it surprising. There are no rules. Girl, you spent over a year having strangers poke you and stick you with needles full of poison. Let this man touch *you*—the real, cancer-free you. Yes, you had cancer. Yes, you have some scars. But you are still a woman. You are a woman who knows how to make love and how to let your mind go so you can enjoy it. It is the most powerful act of reclamation you can make.

12

The Moment
of Truth

Sex after cancer is scary. What will it be like after your numerous chemo treatments and your long sexual drought? Not to mention your new-found vaginal dryness, the beginnings of vaginal atrophy, and a new body that you aren't used to yet. The answer is that it will be as close to being a virgin again as you can get.

You will have fear and trepidation. You will worry that your body will not work the way it is supposed to—the way it used to. And there will be several unknowns circling inside your head: Will I even be able to consummate this act? Will my body hurt so much that I won't be able to continue? Will I repulse my lover because of my scars and my new body? Will he be looking at me and wishing he was with someone else who has not been altered? Will I be able to respond the way I used to? What will it feel like to have my breasts touched?

All these thoughts and others like them not only affect your libido, they affect your self-confidence, as well. We have discussed several things you can do to build up your self-image, and you will be happy you practiced the ways to make you feel and look your best when it comes time to make love for the first time post-cancer.

YOUR PARTNER

Before you and your partner—whoever he may be—begin anything, make sure you are ready. It is important to note that if you have not been practicing any of the exercises previously discussed in this book and if you have excessive dryness and atrophy, having intercourse with your partner could be very painful. Please follow the preparation advice given to you before you attempt sex for the first time. This is a process, and although it takes some work, any obstacle between you and a fulfilling sex life can be overcome. Patience and diligence are the keys. You will get there; you'll see.

Married Women

If your partner is your husband, he has seen the changes to your body take place, and he has witnessed all that you have been through. You two have a history together, even a routine, when it comes to love making. However, the music has now changed and so, too, must your dance steps. This is a learning time; you are going to have to learn the new routines that feel best for you.

Moreover, your husband will be making love to a "new" woman. Not just physically, but mentally, as well. You have changed, my dear, and you should embrace the changes within you because everything that you have endured has made you a stronger, smarter, more intuitive woman, and by extension, lover.

Single Women

If you are single, you have a bit more of a challenge. Dating is hard enough when you have little or nothing serious in your past. But now, you have a medical past that has affected your body, mind, and spirit. It is going to take quite a bit of grit to overcome your anxieties about being with a new man with your new body and the new you.

Here is the question you have to ask yourself: Do you wait for "The One" to make sure everything is in working order? Or, do you resurrect an old lover from your past to help you learn about your new body, so that when "The One" does come along you can truly be the confident, strong, amazing woman that you are?

This is a conscious choice. If you bring back an old boyfriend or a guy you have known for ages who knows you have had cancer and surgeries, make sure you lay everything out on the table first. Use this book as an excuse if you need to. Tell him you are reading a book about sex after cancer, which tells you that you need to get to know the new, sexual you and gain confidence again before you meet the man of your dreams. Offering yourself up to a man with no strings attached is a dream come true for most *men*. However, having sex with someone just to have sex is not easy for many *women*—especially one who is already extremely vulnerable.

There is one rule you must follow before you take on a new lover just for the sake of taking on a lover: Go into it with your eyes wide open. Force yourself to remember that this guy is not looking for anything more than sex from you. If you have never been that kind of girl, this may be very hard to do. Most women, after making love with a man, cannot separate the sex from the feelings. A different organ gets in the way and can turn you into a muddled mess—your heart.

The man who is joining you in the "just for the sex" idea will happily skip along home when it's over and log back on to his Match.com account to resume trolling for new dates. While you, on the other hand, will be remembering tender moments and wondering if maybe, just maybe he fell for you. Don't torture yourself with those thoughts! Remember how you walked into this. It was for the sex only. He does not want you romantically. You may never even see him again. Tell your heart to pipe down and take the experience for what it was—a way to learn about your new body. Heartless? You bet. Doable? Maybe, for some.

Single girls, you may not be made of the stuff it takes to have casual sex. And that is completely understandable. We want to be treasured and loved, so we'd prefer to wait for a man we fall in love with. But as every single woman knows, it may be a long wait. And during that time you'll be constantly wondering how your body will react when "The One" finally comes along and you are intimate with him. So, maybe a trial run isn't such a bad idea?

Whatever you do, think it through. This has to be something you decide for yourself. If you opt for the casual sex route, just keep it in perspective and don't lose sight of what you are really doing. A one night stand can teach you about how your body reacts. But first and foremost, remember to protect your heart. And to use a condom.

PREPARING FOR THE ACT

You will have to prepare yourself for sex. If you have been "training" with toys you will have a pretty good idea about how your body is behaving. But there is a big difference between a toy and a real man. You need to have lubrication at the ready. Display your collection of lubricants and condoms on your bedside table; or, you can store them in a decorative box in a more discreet, but still readily accessible location. Tell your partner that you are not quite sure how your body will respond, so you will have to take it slow and easy.

Get out that lingerie and set the ground rules as to what he can remove and what he cannot remove. Buy long-wear, waterproof makeup and put it over your scars to make them fade if that makes you more confident. If you don't have nipples yet, get the prosthetic, silicone, press-on kind and wear them under your bra. If you have nipples and areolas but have not had your tattoos yet, buy long-wear lipstick in a shade that matches what color your nipples would be and fill in the area with a hint of color. And if you have not had reconstruction, make sure your prosthesis is securely tucked into the pocket of your bra. If you are really worried, buy double-sided wardrobe or toupee tape to secure your bra edges to your skin.

The more you prepare in advance, the less you will have on your mind when the moment comes. Plus, getting these things ready can put you in the mood, which is not a bad thing either! Let's not forget one other thing—*this is fun!* Isn't it about time you started to get yourself some of that?

THE ACT ITSELF

It's time for you to make love. Light a couple of candles in the bedroom. Or, leave the lights on in the other rooms and partially close your bedroom door so there is filtered light coming through—just enough to make things look mysterious and alluring.

Take your time kissing and caressing each other. Move your hands slowly over his body. This will set the speedometer for when he concentrates on your body. Everything you do to him—from kissing to oral sex—should be done at the pace and with the tenderness that you want done on you when it is his turn. If you are worried about not being able to sustain penetration for very long, take a longer time with him orally so he won't take as long to climax during intercourse.

When he turns his attention to you, do not think about how he is kissing you near one of your scars. Remember that he is a man kissing a woman—kissing you. The scars are not important. Try to relax and enjoy each sensation. If he can bring you to orgasm before penetration, you will be far more supple and lubricated. But that is not easy to do the first time with your new body, so talk to him about it beforehand. If you feel very comfortable with him, tell him about your toys. And if he is smart, he will want to use them on you to get you ready. Don't presume he will think of this himself. Men are limited in the imagination department. Gentle suggestions sometimes must become outright requests in order for him to get a clue. But sometimes—as in this case—it's more than worth it.

Penetration

Yikes, he wants in! Will it hurt? Will you bleed? Will you be able to tolerate it? In a word, yes. When he first enters you, you may feel some pain. Make sure you have put on a lot of lube outside and inside your vagina. In fact, have him do it. Even with the lube, though, the first couple of thrusts will be painful. The pain should subside. Remind yourself to relax and you will soon see that your body remembers what to do. With the help of the lube, you will stretch to accommodate him. You may need to be on top so you can control the depth of penetration, and if at anytime you need to stop to add more lubrication, do so. Follow your body's signals, give in to the sensations, and don't forget to breathe.

If the pain does not go away or makes it impossible to continue, you need to revisit the vaginal dilators and topical estrogen conversations with your doctor. You *can* get to a point where you can make love again. You just may need some more help getting there first. Refer back to page 85 for more about this.

Yogic Breathing

If you've ever taken a yoga class, you know that breathing is a very important element of it. Long, cleansing breaths help to keep you centered, and to keep your focus on your body. What you might not know, though, is that the nerves that carry sexual pleasure from the vagina to the brain are the same nerves that are stimulated when you take deep yogic breaths. So, why not apply yoga's breathing principles to our bedrooms?

If you're still not convinced, here's another reason for you. When making love, our minds sometimes wander. We worry about how we look, how he's feeling, and what he's thinking. Then, we worry about climaxing so we hold our breaths and try our hardest. Nothing can ruin your chances of an orgasm more than doing any of those things. Free your mind of everything except what is happening to you physically in that moment. Don't hold your breath. Breathe in and out deeply. Relax. Let your body take over and release completely into the wonderful sensations of lovemaking.

Positions

The missionary position may be a challenge at first because he is on top, meaning he is controlling the force and depth of the thrusts. Instead, take charge and get on top of him. That way you can do what feels best for you. Lay your chest down on his and wrap your feet around his knees. This offers both you and him the best opportunity for stimulation, and it doesn't cause too much trauma to your new body. With each thrust your body will wake up more and more, and if it could talk it would say, "Oh yeah! I remember this. This feels good!"

Another stimulating position that will keep him from going too deep is him on top with his legs open wide, and you on bottom with your legs close together. This makes his body move in areas that will make you feel great once you get going. If you want to try him coming from behind, go beyond the obvious "doggy style." Instead, rest your entire body on the bed and then have him enter you from behind. While this is happening, you can use a vibrator, your hand, or just rub against the bed for added stimulation.

These are just suggestions. With a little experimentation, you will find your best fit and the position that suits you both. You may not even need a bed at all. He could simply sit in a chair and you could straddle him with your legs outstretched. This, too, offers you direct stimulation. The bottom line is that once you discover that yes, indeedy, you can do this, you are only limited by your imagination. Remember, a sexy mind is a terrible thing to waste!

The G-Spot

We have heard a lot about it and some people spend months searching for it. It is the G-spot. When it is finally found and stimulated, it can add a deeper dimension to sex. It has nerve endings that can add to your orgasm and your general, over-all pleasure during lovemaking. The clitoris is still where you will find the most explosive sensations, and ultimately, what will bring you to orgasm. But adding stimulation of the G-spot can increase those feelings and make for an amazing sexual experience.

To find your G-spot, lie down and put a lubricated finger into your vagina with the underside of your finger facing up. Next, bend your finger and press the side of the vaginal wall until you find a tender area. That is the G-spot. Touch it lightly and rhythmically until you find what pleases you. Then, remember the location so you can show it to your man.

Kegels

You have heard that kegel exercises can improve your sex life time and again. But sometimes—as is perhaps the case in this instance—a tip can become so well known that we stop paying attention to it. It is not a new and exciting breakthrough in the enhancement of female pleasure, so it gets ignored. Well, ladies, kegels may not be new, but they work.

The pubococcygeus muscles, or PC muscles, are an integral part of orgasm. They are what contract while a woman is climaxing. The stronger those muscles are, the better the woman's ability to reach orgasm, and the orgasm itself, will be.

Where are they and how do you locate them? The easiest way to locate your PC muscles and to feel them working is to stop your urine flow mid-stream. The muscles that allow you to do that are the PC muscles. To get an idea of how they are effective sexually, insert a lubricated finger into your vagina and contract those muscles. You will feel a tightening sensation, and you will also feel pleasure.

If you build up the strength of these muscles, you can help bring about an orgasm during lovemaking just by tightening and releasing them while your partner is inside you. And when you do finally reach orgasm, it will be much stronger than before. The best part is that you can strengthen your PC muscles anywhere—while driving your kids to school, standing on line at the post office, or sitting here reading this book. Simply tighten the muscle for three seconds, hold for three seconds, then release. Do this ten times a day and in about a month you will notice a difference. You will feel more vaginal sensation during intercourse and you will be able to help bring on an orgasm. Then, when you do climax with strong PC muscles, it will be memorable!

Orgasm

The best time for you to reach orgasm is before penetration. If you don't, it may be hard to get there during intercourse the first couple of times. That's okay. You don't have to reach orgasm to have great sex. If your partner is a good lover, he will know you didn't get there. And any man worth his salt should know that if you did not climax, that he should offer to bring you there after he has finished. It is just plain bad manners not to!

If men only knew what this little step could do for their street credibility as lovers, they would do it a lot more. However, the truth of the matter is that it's sometimes up to us to teach them. Don't lie there languishing. If he is not a jerk and doesn't roll over and start snoring immediately, take his hand, put it between your legs, and simply whisper, "my turn." If he does not help you get there after that, then you really need to re-examine this guy and your future together. Seriously.

SEXUAL ETIQUETTE

We've come a long way, baby—a long way from the Victorian days of yore where sex education for women consisted of telling them to "lie back and think of England." But we have gone off the track a bit, too. The sexual revolution of the 1960s and 70s set new rules. Mainly, that anything goes. That is fine if you don't care about your heart or lasting memories. But if you do, you should still follow some basic rules of sexual etiquette. There are some for your partner to follow, as well.

Rules for You

- Do not presume he can read your mind.

- Do not believe you can change him or make him love you.

- Stubble is never okay. Even if you have been married for fifty years, shave your legs, your underarms, and anywhere else that is unruly.

- A man who calls you for a date after ten at night wants sex and nothing more.

- The Internet is a good tool to make sure you're not dating a serial killer, but it is not okay to use it to cyberstalk your date. By all means Google him so you know he is who he says he is, but stalking him and his friends on Facebook is one step away from Bunny Boiler territory.

- After a date, never email, text, Twitter, phone, or send a smoke signal before he does. Don't do it. We have spoiled men rotten with this. When one comes along that is truly interested, he will woo *you*.

- Always use protection. Never believe what he says, because some men will say anything to have sex without a condom.

- Just because he bought you dinner does not mean he bought you. You do not owe him anything.

- Wear underwear.

- Be honest when making love. Otherwise, he will think he knows what he is doing and you won't ever be able to get satisfied. If he doesn't get you there, tell him. Do not fake it unless you just want to get it over with. Note, though, that if you just want to get it over with, it may be a clue that he is not the man for you.

Rules for Your Partner

- You are not too busy to keep up with your personal hygiene. If you can't shower before a date, invest in baby wipes. Skid marks may be acceptable to your tighty whities, but they'll gross us out beyond imagination.

- No, you are not that big, so please don't ask us to elaborate on the issue. We will coo, ooo, and ahh, but for the love of God don't ever tell us about how women are "intimidated" by your girth. Please. If you are straight, we have seen more erections than you have.

- We are not potholes and do not require the jackhammer treatment . . . unless we ask for it.

- Don't try every position you can think of the first time we make love. You are not in Cirque de Soliel. Concentrate on what gives us pleasure instead of showing off.

- We have as much of a right to reach orgasm as you do. If we don't get there, offer to help us after you are done. We talk, and trust us, you don't want that rap.

- Tell us we are beautiful, even if we look like Ernest Borgnine. Lie if you have to. Just make us feel desirable.

- Email, text, phone, or Twitter us the next day so we don't feel completely used.

- Be honest. If you are a player, let us know upfront. That way we don't torment ourselves thinking we can make you love us.

- If you are married, go home to your wife and leave us alone.

- Show emotion. It won't kill you. No woman wants to make love to a Vulcan.

Current society would have us believe that there may be something to reducing your carbon footprint by not shaving your legs. And he may foolishly think he can be a total jerk because he is "so great" and can still get girls. But long-term, meaningful relationships aren't built that way. Once you get over your fears and realize you can, indeed, make love again, make love for *real*. Don't settle for anything less than a wonderful experience. Make your man step up to the plate if he is lacking, or reassure him so he can live up to his full potential. If he is not what you are looking for, cut him loose and find someone else. If he is everything you ever dreamed of, hold on tight. As John Lennon once said, "And in the end, the love you take, is equal to the love you make."

13

Free Your Mind and Body

Your life, post-cancer, has its victories and its fears. Surviving is, of course, a victory. But the truth is that you still feel sheer terror at every new monitoring or regular test. It is normal to be afraid that something will be found again. After all, it already happened to you once and that is hard to forget. Your imagination has probably written a whole new playbook; every headache is a brain tumor, every cough becomes lung cancer, and on and on. We have all been there.

It's time to give yourself permission to be well, though. The day-to-day battle against this disease is over. Reprogram your mind to live in relative peace, and stop projecting into the future with a million "what ifs." Worrying is normal, but spending every moment thinking your cancer will come back won't get you anywhere. Life is a beautiful collection of moments—moments that are never repeated the same way again. Do you want to spend your days missing those moments because you are preoccupied by the anxiety that your cancer will return? Or, do you want to be present in every second, living your life to its fullest? Cherish every moment you have—you fought long and hard for each one of them.

Your cancer has been removed surgically, chemically, and radioactively. You are about to start your life as a true survivor, doing your best to remain that way forever. Living, *really* living, is knowing that right here, right now, in this moment, you are alive. Live your life with joy, and don't ever let fear take over or rob you of that joy. If you do, cancer wins. Piss cancer off and live well—don't let it interfere with your life. That is the best revenge. Yes, you will feel positively awful some days. You will feel tired and crappy and want to cry all the time. So, make your good days count. Do not let the Beast in because that is what it wants. You have survived your cancer, now start living. When someone asks you about your situation, don't say, "I have cancer." Instead say, "I am a survivor" and believe it. Because that's exactly what you are.

To reinforce the positive, keep a journal by your bed. Before you turn off the light and go to sleep each night, count the blessings you experienced that day. Keep negative thoughts out. Just write the good things that make you happy and bring you peace. Then, close the journal, turn off the light, and go to sleep with your blessings on your mind. Worry and stress are not allowed, only good things.

POST-TRAUMATIC STRESS AND DEPRESSION

The most misunderstood and under-acknowledged long-term side effect of cancer has no scan or x-ray to show its damage. No, this side effect is psychological, and it is a wound that many patients bear. Some find a way to cope with it and go on living their lives. But more do not.

The unfortunate truth is that many survivors who go back to see their oncologists for a check-up two or three years out of treatment are severely depressed. Their friends and relatives are often amazed by this. How can they be depressed? They survived cancer! Nevertheless, feelings of hopelessness, despair, loneliness, and heartbreak persist. They cannot concentrate. They either don't sleep, or sleep too much. They lose interest in life and participate in fewer and fewer activities. They are, quite literally, shadows of their former selves.

Why? Before the world jumps in with talk of antidepressants and therapy, the "why" must be examined. A breast cancer patient has watched the life she knew get pulled out from under her. She has been betrayed by her own body, and what was once safe and familiar has become the enemy. She endured the treatments, was told how wonderful and strong she is, and was then abruptly shoved back into her life.

What life, though? The healthy, carefree, pre-cancer girl's life is gone. The brave warrior in constant battle-mode has completed her tour of duty. And the upbeat trooper enduring everything with a smile needs a break. She is tired. And now she is expected to seamlessly return to her pre-cancer life and simultaneously accommodate the new woman she has become. Daunting? You bet. Overwhelming? Absolutely.

This is, in fact, a form of post-traumatic stress disorder. As cancer patients, we were so busy fighting that we were just going through the motions of life. We spent so much energy hoping that when "real life" kicked back in, things would indeed change for the better. Unfortunately, along the way we forgot to acknowledge how all of this affected our souls. Our wounds go beyond the physical. Our hearts were broken. The entire time we were trying to be strong and brave, the little girl inside of us was terrified and just wanted to hide. So, when we are "all done" and supposed to snap out of it and return to exactly where we were before this disease, we can't. We simply aren't the same people anymore.

When we are down and out like this, we can't see how beautiful and strong we have become. The months go by and we faithfully visit our physicians for check-ups and terror-filled scans to be sure the cancer has not returned. Until one day we notice it. We are just going through the motions. Nothing is real. And that is when the depression can catch us.

This is a big problem that the medical community must address. Just like soldiers who have served their country, survived battles, and are then simply sent home when the war is over, breast cancer survivors are shipped back home with little more than a pat on the head. Doctors tell them to go live their lives, but they forget to treat one very important thing—the spirit.

Your spirit helped you stay in fight-mode throughout your treatments. It has borne the effects of your surgeries and chemotherapy sessions, and the brunt of the ice-cold fear every exam and blood test brings. Because of this, your spirit has never had the opportunity to heal. And until it does, you may not feel that you have truly survived.

You must acknowledge this. You can't wait for a doctor to *maybe* pick up on a change in your demeanor. Once your body has healed, your life must heal, your spirit must be thanked for its strength and courage, and then it must be given a break. This is a rough road we have traveled. Again, like any warrior returning from battle, you have scars you see and scars you don't see. A reconditioning must occur, and a loving respite must be given to your weary spirit.

Does feeling depressed in any way diminish your success? Absolutely not. It is part of the process. But it would help if more doctors were aware—and subsequently made their patients aware—that this feeling is normal. If feeling better means taking a course of antidepressants, then do it. Do whatever it is you have to do to feel safe and at home with yourself again.

When it comes down to it, you are the only one who can really help yourself, but that is hard when you are feeling hopeless and helpless. If you are finding this to be true, try this exercise. Imagine a little girl who has been through something really scary. She is in a dark room and she is surrounded by adults. No one hears her. She is trying to get noticed. She is desperately looking for a way out—for a way home where she can be safe and happy again. Now imagine you are one of the adults in the room with the little girl. Your heart cries out to her. You scoop her up in your arms and carry her out into the sunshine. As you walk together, the mist clears and she can see her house and her familiar surroundings in the distance. She starts to feel safe again, and she feels joy that she is home.

The little girl is you. The adult is also you. That is how we take care of ourselves. Now is the time to take care of *you*. If you see you are in a dark and scary place, take the steps to free yourself and go to the light—to the joy. Carry yourself back home.

SELF ESTEEM

Accept the following concept: You are a work of art, not a science project. Art is lovingly created. It takes time, and it shows. People treasure works of art and want to be near them. Treasure who you are and who you have become. Free your body, mind, and soul from the cold, impersonal exam rooms you frequented on a regular basis in the past. You are not what used to be, you are what will be. And you are free now. Free to be whomever you want to be. Some cancer survivors even say that every day is their birthday. Each new day is one day farther away from diagnosis, and is therefore a celebration of life. And they do indeed celebrate it. Getting to that point begins by reconnecting with your body and focusing on what you can change. Think of it as a birthday present to yourself.

Reconnect with Your Body

You have come out of your cancer treatments with a new body. Whether you reconstructed or not, it's new. Many times, women who do reconstruct do not feel connected to their new breasts. There is a term for them that many survivors use, which is *"foobs,"* for fake boobs. This is not a good way to look at a brand new part of your anatomy. Your boobs are yours. They may still be under construction, but there should not be a disconnect between you and them. You have to accept them into the family. And stop calling them *foobs*! If you must call them something other than breasts, at least call them *"noobs,"* because that more accurately describes what they are—your new boobs.

And what if you didn't reconstruct? You may have felt a shock to your system when you first looked at yourself without breasts. But remember, you chose not to reconstruct and there was a reason for that. Usually, when a woman chooses to forego reconstruction it is because she has very healthy self esteem, and she sees herself as more than just her breasts. At least that was the idea at the time of surgery . . .

Maybe now you are questioning your decision. Don't worry. You can always get breasts if you want to. But do you really want to? If you still feel as confident as you did when you made your choice and you are happy with your decision to stay au natural, revel in it! The legend of the Amazons is that they removed their breasts so they would not get in the way of their bows and arrows as they fought off their enemies. What could be a stronger symbol than that? On the other hand, there is also something delicately feminine about an unreconstructed breast. Remember Degas' paintings of precious ballerinas that we spoke of earlier? None of them have any breasts to speak of, yet they are some of the loveliest depictions of the female form that can be found.

The bottom line is that whether or not you chose to reconstruct, own it. Make the best out of what you have. And remember, nothing is set in stone. Your surgical site is not a final sale, so if you don't like how your breasts look, tell your plastic surgeon you want a do-over. You have many options, so do whatever you need to in order to feel satisfied with your appearance.

Focus on What You Can Change

When you once again begin to feel connected to your body, your next task is to find a way to make yourself feel *comfortable* in it. This can be accomplished in many ways, but a great place to start is with exercise. Watch your body change as it gets stronger. Feel the muscles in your thighs after a long bike ride. Take a yoga class to center yourself—breathe in peace and acceptance, and breathe out all that built up stress and anxiety you accumulated during treatment.

If you had low self esteem before cancer, having your body altered forever can be almost unbearable. Hopefully you have read the parts of this book that show you how to look great and feel even better about yourself. (If not, turn to page 41 immediately!) Put your body issues into perspective. All women have figure flaws and everyone has something that they hate about themselves. However, it is how we perceive those imperfections that really makes or breaks how we feel about ourselves.

There are things about your body that you can change, but be realistic about what they are. For example, don't stress over the fact that you are 5'1". You aren't going to change that so you might as well stop obsessing about wanting to be taller. On the other hand, if you don't like having grey hair, a change is only a salon trip away. Similarly, your plastic surgeon can give you liposuction in those saddle-bags that you hate, and then transfer the fat to the marionette lines on your face that you hate. Talk about a win-win situation! You found two things you wanted to change and one procedure that can handle both. When getting down on yourself, try to remember the mantra: "Every problem has a solution." This is true of all the things you know you actually *can* change about yourself.

Before you decide on any procedure, though, test your view of yourself to make sure you aren't "seeing" things that no one else does. There are two ways you can do this. The first is to stand in front of a mirror so that you cannot see your face—only your body. Now that you are detached from your body, look at it as if it is the body of a stranger. What are the things you like? What are the things you don't like? Divide the things you don't like into those you can improve and those that you were born with. Then, move forward by conquering what you can change and doing your best to come to terms with what you can't.

The second way we have already used in the previous chapter to see how we looked—*really* looked—in jeans. Do the same thing now. Take your camera and put it on self timer. Stand in front of it in your underwear and capture all angles of yourself. Then, download all of them onto your computer and crop them so that you cannot see your head. Is your butt really as big as you think it is? Are your arms really that flabby? Chances are they are not. When we get down on ourselves, we literally see our bodies in a distorted way. But when we see a faceless photograph, we can evaluate ourselves more objectively. Again, from this exercise decide if there is an area you still want to improve. If it is something that can be done, find a way to improve it.

It is important to note that some of us are so paralyzed by a negative self image that nothing, not even these simple exercises, can help. If you still feel truly bad about yourself, find someone to talk to. You don't need to be depressed to get therapy. Seeking help for a poor body image is just as important, and it is the course you need to take.

COUNSELING

There is no reason to suffer. If breast cancer isn't a legitimate enough reason to send a person into therapy, then what is? Working through your problems, fears, and doubts will go a long way toward healing your spirit. It is healthy to talk to someone about all the emotions that you held in while you were being so strong for everyone else. There are all levels of counseling and counselors, and the following information may help you select which kind is right for you.

Live Groups

There are groups for breast cancer survivors that meet in person. These can be good while you are in treatment, but they can also be scary because they are comprised of people in all stages of their disease. If you have stage one cancer, what you are going through is a lot different than what someone living with metastatic disease is going through. You are freaked out about the future, and the metastatic survivor is freaked out about freaking everyone else out, so she feels she can't express her true feelings. For this reason, these groups don't always work. If you can find one that is specific to your stage and where you are in your journey, that is the best way to go. Otherwise, be careful. They may do more harm than good.

Online Groups

There are many online support groups both for women with breast cancer and for women living after breast cancer. The benefits of online groups are that you can lurk and just read what other women are saying, jump in when you want, be with people from all over the world, and wake up in the middle of the night and know that someone will be there. Additionally, you can do it all in your pajamas— your *very stylish* pajamas, of course! You can find a wonderful group of women who are in all stages of breast cancer—from the newly diagnosed to the long term survivor—at www.nosurrenderbreast-cancerfoundation.org, and there is a list of other online groups in the resource section (page 203). You can learn a lot from your fellow sisters, and communicating with them through an online forum is both liberating and comforting at the same time.

Social Workers

Another way to find help is with a social worker who has a master's degree. Look for one who specializes in women with breast cancer. Often, they have small groups that meet in their offices, too. If you can find someone who has been through breast cancer herself, it would be ideal. It can be hard to speak to someone who can't personally relate to your issues. It really takes a survivor to get what it is you are going through. If your social worker has not experienced breast cancer firsthand, mention to her that you are concerned that she may not understand your true feelings. The two of you can then work through that so there are no barriers between you.

Psychologists

Psychologists may have more advanced degrees than social workers and they may be more of what you are looking for, simply because their advanced degrees give them a wider scope of understanding and resources. Additionally, some, but not all, are covered by insurance plans. Contact your provider to see what type of mental health services you are covered for, and who is in your particular plan.

Psychiatrists

Psychiatrists are medical doctors that specialize in psychiatry. They can write prescriptions for medications that may help you, and they may have a better understanding of the chemical changes that have occurred as a result of your treatment. You have a better chance of your insurance covering a psychiatrist than you do with the other counseling professionals because they are medical doctors.

The first step is for you to accept that you may need some outside help to overcome the emotional toll your cancer took on you. Speak

to your oncologist or primary care physician and ask them for recommendations. This will make your search to find the right professional for you a little easier. You may have to "test drive" a couple
before you find the perfect fit, but once you feel comfortable with
someone, get to work. And counseling *is* work. You may have to
dredge up some unpleasant feelings before you can start to feel better again, but this uncomfortable process is well worth the end result.

PRE-EXISTING CONDITIONS
THAT TAKE OVER AFTER CANCER

Sometimes conditions that you didn't know you had before suddenly flare up after cancer treatment. Since chemotherapy affects
your immune system, your ability to ward off these conditions is
weakened. Many women discover that the little touch of arthritis
they had before cancer is more severe after chemotherapy. Some put
the blame on hormonal treatments and the lack of estrogen, but it
may just be a simple arthritic flare. This is why it is important to keep
your primary care physician in the loop of all you are going through
during and after cancer treatment.

There are several other things you should keep an eye on now
that your treatments are over, like your thyroid. Your thyroid can
change after radiation. If your hair is not growing back or is sparse,
if you have dry skin, if you feel lethargic, or if you cannot lose
weight, get your thyroid level checked. In addition, your cholesterol
can become elevated from certain hormonal treatments, so make sure
you have it checked, as well. Migraines may be made worse by the
sudden drop in estrogen and blood pressure may also become elevated, so be sure to get both levels checked.

Three things you should absolutely not neglect post-treatment
are your ovaries, your uterus, and your colon. Many doctors suggest
removing your ovaries to help lower your estrogen level even more
than the hormonal treatment already is. If you are on Tamoxifen, you
must make frequent visits to your gynecologist to check your uterine
lining. It can build up while you're on that drug, which can sometimes, on rare occasions, cause pre-cancerous cells to grow. You also

need to watch for blood clots if you are on Tamoxifen. Please speak to your doctor about this.

Finally, if you have never had a colonoscopy before, now is the time to get one. The procedure is done in one day, and it's quick and easy. The day before when you have to "clean out" is not fun, but after chemo, it is child's play. Studies have shown that there is a link between breast cancer and colorectal cancer. The good news is that colon cancer is preventable if the growths are found early through colonoscopy screening, so getting it done is a good insurance policy.

FEMALE SEXUAL DYSFUNCTION— INABILITY TO REACH ORGASM

If you are having trouble reaching orgasm, you are not alone. According to a recent study from the *Journal of the American Medical Association*, 43 percent of women cannot reach orgasm. So rest assured, it's not just you and it's not just the cancer. The technical term for the inability to climax is female sexual dysfunction, and there are many factors that contribute to it.

However, if this is something new to you and only started happing after your diagnosis, you *can* blame it on cancer. At the 2009 San Antonio Breast Cancer Symposium, Memorial Sloan-Kettering Center in New York released data from a two-year study. It concluded that, "Sexual dysfunction is prevalent in women treated for breast cancer and should be discussed with patients as a potential adverse effect of therapy. Assessment of sexual symptoms throughout treatment and beyond may facilitate the use of potential interventions such as lubricants, dilators, treatment modification, topical estrogens, and counseling."

What Causes Female Sexual Dysfunction?

Most medical books state two reasons for female sexual dysfunction. The first is that a woman has never had an orgasm in her life. The second is that because of some trauma, she can no longer reach orgasm. The medical books all lean heavily on the psychological reasons a woman cannot reach climax, more so than focusing on the physical causes.

To find out if your problem is psychological or physical, you need to see if you can bring about an orgasm by yourself. If you can, and you only have problems when you are with a man, then physically there is nothing wrong with you, which means you can rule that out. However, it also means that you need to work on your psychological ability to orgasm with a man. If you find that the exercises discussed earlier in this book bring you pleasure but that you cannot recreate that with your partner, the two of you may need couple's or sex therapy, which will give the two of you exercises to do together.

The best way for a woman to reach orgasm with a man is through long foreplay and a great deal of oral sex. You need to speak candidly to your partner about this. Tell him constructively by saying something like, "When you go down on me you make me crazy. Can you stay there longer? I really love it!" Then, if he does do this and you feel yourself ready to climax, don't stop. Go for it and have an orgasm. Many women, when they are almost there during oral sex, stop their partner and pull them up so that intercourse can begin. This may be a very passionate gesture, but for some women it is like turning off the engine. They then have to restart it again and try to build back up from there.

If you can orgasm while receiving oral sex from your partner, do it! It really is the best thing you can do, because then when you start intercourse your nerve endings will be on fire, you will be supple and lubricated, and the chances of you reaching another orgasm are great. Additionally, if you have practiced your Kegels and use them while all of this is happening, you will find intercourse to be absolutely amazing.

If talking it out and experimenting with your partner doesn't work, you really must get help for this. Find a professional you trust and work it out. You should not live your life missing out on pleasure.

Common Libido Drains

If your problem is in fact physical, not psychological, first take a look at the medications you are on. If you find that they can keep you from reaching orgasm, speak to your doctor about switching. Take an especially close look at your antidepressants if you are on them, as they may be affecting your libido. Traditionally, Selective Serotonin Re-Uptake Inhibitors (SSRI's) are the biggest culprits. Effexor is one such drug. While many women find that it helps reduce hot flashes, it also reduces sexual response and desire. There are other drugs, like Wellbutrin, that do not have this side effect, so be sure to talk to your doctor about alternative options.

Another factor that can affect your sexual desire is being in early menopause, either from chemotherapy or from having to shut down your ovaries. Menopause drastically reduces the estrogen level in your body, thus explaining the diminished desire. It can also lead to physical changes that may make sexual activity painful. However, those physical changes are all reversible. Really!

Chapter 6 (page 75) provides some good suggestions to get you through this initial pain, but there are other products made specifically for women that you should also know about. One is called Zestra and the other is KY Intense. They are formulated with ingredients such as evening primrose oil, angelica root, coleus forskohlii extract, vitamin E, and natural fragrances. When applied, they increase sensitivity to the vaginal area, as well as promote arousal, sensation, and the ability to reach orgasm.

However, if your tissues are thin and hypersensitive, it can cause burning and pain, so it is best to take it for a test drive on your own before you try it with your partner. That being said, if you are not sensitive to its ingredients, it is like a hit of Red Bull for your vagina. It will wake up all of your nerve endings, making your entire vaginal area very responsive. Speaking of Red Bull, caffeine helps increase feeling and sexual response after you drink it, as well. Who knew?

Lubricants

We already discussed lubricants a little earlier, but they're important to mention again here because they can help make sex possible—thereby helping you reach orgasm. New products are being introduced every day as more and more women demand them. For instance, KY makes a liquid bead that you can insert hours before sex. It looks like a big jelly bean and comes with an applicator. After insertion, the outer shell dissolves and you are left completely moisturized and lubricated for as many as three days. Products like this allow you to keep a little spontaneity in your sex life, and end the need to stop in the middle of foreplay to add lube—both things that may help you reach orgasm.

In addition to KY's liquid beads, there are also silicone-based lubricants that are very long-lasting. They do not bead up like some of the water-soluble lubricants do, either. One of the most popular, and most expensive, is Pjur from Germany. A little goes a long way. And since it is so long lasting, you can apply it long before you go to the bedroom.

Another product some women swear by is coconut oil. This can be great, but it can also be messy. It comes in a solidified form, but it quickly melts in your fingers and makes a slippery mess of everything. There is a way to avoid that, though. In fact, you can use this tip universally for all the lubrication products you wish to try. Use a syringe. Get a large syringe, without the needle, of course, from your doctor or pharmacy. Fill it up with your lubricant of choice and then lie on your back and "inject" it inside your vagina. This puts it in place and gets you ready for action later on. It is also a particularly great idea for coconut oil lovers, specifically, because it stays solidified until it is inside you, which eliminates the mess.

Do whatever you need to do to get your mind and your body ready for sex. Once you do, you will free yourself to the pleasures of orgasm. It will take some work, some "heart" work, for you to step out of the shadows of your past and into the light again, but you can do it. You have been through a lot and all that trauma has built up around you in layers. You must peel each layer off now, one at a time, to free yourself. As mentioned earlier, it is a process, but it is so worth it.

14

$\mathscr{L}$ove

ove. What a beautiful word. What a beautiful concept—especially after hearing that you may die. Tennessee Williams once said, "At the other end of death, is love." Cancer shows us how to love deeper and truer than we ever have before. How could it not? We now know what is real, we know what matters, and we no longer settle. Whether you are married or single, you will find yourself wanting a deeper kind of love in your life. Look for it both in yourself and in others, and don't ever give up looking, because it is out there.

FAMILIAL LOVE

If you thought you had a close family before cancer, it is undoubtedly even closer now. And if there were rifts in certain relationships before, all that pettiness now seems foolish. You've seen, firsthand, that life is very unpredictable, so now is as good a time as any to bring everyone together again. This Thanksgiving, have the whole family over for dinner at your house—even the people who don't get along with each other. If they grumble when you invite them, pull the cancer card and say, "I just finished chemotherapy for cancer. I want the whole family together." Go ahead and use guilt as your ally, because in this instance, you are using it for good. Then, when you see your family members all around you—your life all around you—tell them you love them and celebrate the moment. Remember, you are a moment collector now. And family gatherings are doozies.

Why is family so important? Because they knew you "when." They knew you when you would race around the backyard screaming after your brothers, and they knew you when you got that scar on your knee that needed twelve stitches. You and your family have been through joyful and sad times together. They still see you as the sister or daughter you were, and it breaks their hearts to think of you going through all that you have. However, when you show them that just like that knee of yours, you may have a scar but your cancer is also a thing of the past, they can see that you are still *you* and life can finally return to normal.

If you have kids of your own, your whole family had to hit the pause button for awhile. Now you are back and you are all moving forward together. Remember that cancer didn't just happen to you. It happened to your family, too. And because of that, you are all stronger and appreciate each other all the more. Love does conquer all. So, too, does joy. Don't let cancer rob you and your family of another moment of joy.

ROMANTIC LOVE

It is possible to find true love after cancer. If you are married, you may find yourself falling in love with your husband all over again. Your battle with cancer terrified him, and his love for you was buried with worry and fear. He has dreamed of the day when he would get you back and it has finally arrived. Because you have opened yourself up to life again, he is free to feel all those old feelings of love and romance. This could be a beautiful chapter in both of your lives. All of the excitement of your early days together can be rekindled. You will be discovering each other's bodies like new lovers. This time, stay lovers as well as husband and wife. Don't lose that magical feeling ever again.

Single survivor, your life is just beginning. You have a world of hope and love ahead of you. You believed in love before, and now you should believe in it even more. Cancer may not be what you had planned. After all, the princesses in story books don't get mastectomies. But stop waiting for the storybook ending. Make a better ending all on your own. While it may not be what you had dreamed of, it could be even better if the love you find is true, deep, and real.

Yes, things are a mess when you get right down to it. You will have to explain your cancer history to your dates and hope that they will take you for who you are. But you have to take that chance or you will never know! Love won't change your cancer past. But it can overcome it and it is worth the ride. Heck, it is worth the price of admission alone! Take that chance. Don't wait for perfect to come find you. Get out there and find him.

SELF LOVE

If you don't love yourself, how do you expect anyone else to love you? This is not trite. It is real. If you have a secret self-loathing of your body and yourself because of what you have been through, it will show.

Have you ever sat back and thought, "Holy crap, I did it. I survived cancer and look at me now. I am okay!"? The strength that carried you through this mess is gorgeous. Be proud of yourself. Love both who you are and who you were. You may have been raised to not brag or boast. You may have hidden your light under a bushel your whole life. Well, honey, you have had radiation now. You are glowing and you can't hide your awesome light anymore.

Write down a list of all of your good qualities if it helps you to see your light. Include all the things you do for others and all the things you do well. Look in the mirror and smile, and then list all of your features you love. List everything you have overcome this past year, too. Now read the list—over and over again.

Look at you! Look at who you are. You did it, girl. You are a survivor. How can you not love you?

LET GO OF YOUR FEARS ABOUT THE FUTURE

Do you find that you often hesitate to take steps forward because you are afraid of the future? Do you say no to going out on a date with a man because you don't want him to have to deal with your cancer? Do you avoid making plans with your husband because you are afraid to think too far in advance for anything? These are all normal emotions, but you can't stop living. You have to release yourself from the prison that fear has kept you in. When you do, you will once again feel excited about life and you will love to plan things.

Let go. No one knows what the future will bring. People who don't have cancer die suddenly. Their futures were just as tenuous as you think yours is now. The only difference is that they didn't spend their lives holding back, because they had no clue that some horrible thing was going to strike them down. They lived their lives. They lived lives free of fear of the future and they made plans. It is time for you to think like that. Think like a cancer-free person. Think like a survivor.

LET GO OF MEN WHO WON'T COMMIT OUT OF FEAR FOR YOUR FUTURE

Some men are idiots. They don't want to get serious with you or stay in your marriage because they are afraid you will get sick again. Do they have a crystal ball? Can they tell which women will and will not get breast cancer in their lifetimes? The average now is that one in seven women will be diagnosed at some point in their lives. So, there is a one in seven chance that the "healthy" woman he leaves you for will also get breast cancer. What will he do then? Leave her too?

If you have that type of man in your life—one who hesitates because he isn't quite sure you are going to make it, thereby making you a burden to him and his precious plans—you do not want him. If you get that signal from a man, dump him. He is nothing but fair-weathered and his negativity will drain you. Heaven help him if something untoward should ever happen to him!

PERSONAL STORY: JILL DOESN'T MAKE THE CUT

Jill is a successful health care professional who also happens to be a breast cancer survivor. She is single, forty-five, and beautiful. She has a great life and dates occasionally, but she really hasn't met "The One" yet. The last man she dated was actually one of her doctors, which she found to be a relief! After all, he already knew everything about her medical history, and a man in medicine does not need breast cancer explained to him. She thought she would finally be able to relax.

They met for dinner and had a nice date. She didn't have to talk about her cancer. In fact, she really didn't get a chance to talk much at all. He was too busy talking about himself and his general unhappiness with world affairs for her to get a word in edgewise. Nonetheless, they had a second date and she invited him to her house for coffee. During their conversation, he told Jill—in general terms—that no doctor would get serious with someone who had cancer because all people with cancer die. Although he never referred to himself specifically, his intent was still made abundantly clear. He went on to tell her that no doctor wants to deal with that because they know how dreadful it is at the end.

Jill sat there in stunned amazement as she realized what an utter asshole this guy was. He left soon after those comments were made, and she did not hear from him again until three months later when she had a follow-up appointment with him as her doctor. When he walked into the exam room, he hugged her and said, "The reason I dumped you is because I was diagnosed with prostate cancer." Jill wanted to correct him and tell him that he never had her to begin with so she wasn't his to dump, but it didn't matter. She also restrained herself from sarcastically telling him that women don't want to get serious with men who had prostate cancer because it's just "so dreadful."

Despite her urges, she took the high road and wished him all the best. Jill knew she didn't have to say a word to this man—Karma had taken care of him for her. And never in her life had she seen Karma work so fast! As she was leaving his office with his instructions to come back again in another three months, she asked his receptionist for copies of her medical records and found herself a new doctor.

Today, Jill's old doctor is cancer-free and doing fine. He is still single. Jill, on the other hand, is in love with a wonderful architect who adores her.

LONG-TERM PLANS ARE REALISTIC

Was the doctor right? Is it unrealistic for a breast cancer survivor to make long-term plans with a man? No! Ladies, Jill's doctor couldn't have been more wrong. His life didn't end because of his prostate cancer. He got treated, kept practicing medicine, and is still dating. Your life will go on, too!

Maybe this experience taught Jill's doctor not to be so heartless, but unfortunately, having cancer doesn't instantly make you a better person. Sometimes people become angry, bitter, and hopeless. They are the ones who don't make long-term plans and dwell in negative places. Don't let yourself become one of these people. You have your whole life ahead of you. Make as many plans as you can fit into it. Suck the pap out of life. Get a thirty year loan. Invest in a retirement plan. Don't live like you are dying, remember?

BROKEN HEARTS

Having cancer doesn't make you immune from people being cruel to you or breaking your heart. In fact, you might find that certain relationships you thought you'd have forever have started to crumble. Friends may have become flaky. If you are married, your husband may have showed you his true colors, which weren't pretty. And if you are single, men don't suddenly become Knights in shining armor.

Be your own Knight. Remember who you are and all that you have overcome. You have quite a bit of courage inside you. You have courage to move away from toxic people, and courage to take chances you never thought you would before cancer.

When you break a bone, it grows back stronger than it was before. Similarly, a breast cancer diagnosis may break our spirit, our sense of security, and our sense of self. It takes awhile for us to heal from that, but once we do, we are stronger, more resilient people.

Anytime we are faced with something frightening we can say to ourselves, "Hell, I did chemo. That can't scare me." If friends hurt us, we can clean them out. Cancer taught us that life is too short to let negative people drain us of our hope and our newfound good feelings. Negativity is also counterproductive to the healing process. Stress can cause all sorts of diseases, so we move away from those who mean us harm. And that includes the men in our lives . . .

There is a danger of staying in a relationship—a bad relationship—too long because we feel we can't do any better. We see our partners as men who are "willing" to be with us and tell ourselves we shouldn't look a gift horse in the mouth. This happens quite frequently to women who have not yet come to terms with their new bodies and new lives. Eventually, they realize that they are worth more than the way they are being treated. They realize that they are the gifts in the relationship, not the other way around.

If you find yourself putting up with a situation that you would never have tolerated before cancer, step back and reevaluate the situation. Do you love him more than you love yourself? If the answer is no—if you love yourself more than you love him—get out and find a new love. There is new love out there. Don't stay in a toxic situation because you think you won't ever find someone else to love; you will if you try.

If, on the other hand, he is the one who leaves you and you feel like you won't ever be happy again, think back to how you felt when you were first diagnosed. That was almost certainly the worst time of the whole cancer experience. Everything was new, foreign, and terrifying. You never thought you would make it through the next week, much less the next year. But you did. You can handle heartache. Follow the advice in the beginning of this book. The cure for men is more men! Don't lock yourself away because you don't have one anymore. Get out there and find another!

GIVE YOURSELF PERMISSION TO BE HAPPY

Give yourself the gift of happiness and do whatever it takes to keep it. How do you give yourself happiness? Take a look around. Do you like where you live? Do you like how it looks? Make your surroundings beautiful and have them reflect your personal style. Put things in your home and garden that you love. If you always wanted to have a bedroom painted Tiffany Box blue with crisp white curtains and a matching duvet, what's stopping you? Even if your husband tells you he prefers a beige, plaid bedspread, do it anyway.

Plant a cutting garden so you always have fresh flowers in your home in the summer. Start to entertain more. Married women, this is a good way for you and your husband to be seen as a happy, healthy, fun-loving team again, instead of that couple whose wife had cancer. Single women, throwing a dinner party is a great way to meet men. How? Invite a core group of your friends, as well as one or two single men that you know and may want to get to know better. It is a non-threatening situation for all involved because it is a party with several people, not just the two of you. There isn't any first date weirdness. Instead, he will see you as a funny, happy woman who knows how to throw a great party. Moreover, having two single men there will spark their competition gene, so don't be surprised if you end up with two dates the next weekend!

When people are diagnosed with cancer, it is like they have been dreaming their whole lives and suddenly they are awakened. You had a wake-up call and now the best of your life awaits you. Breathe in the new air and see the world come alive around you. Where once you only scratched the surface of your potential, you now see it is time to swing for the fences. Take the time to make yourself feel good. Make that extra effort to dress nicely. Go get your hair done. Wear fantastic lingerie-every day. Take the long way home and stop along the way at a shop or pub you've always wanted to go to. Say I love you—to others and to yourself.

A lot was asked of you—and a lot was lost to you—because of cancer. But you have also gained more from this experience than you probably ever imagined. Now it is your turn to control your own life. It's your world—your way. The first chance you took was on the day you were born. Why stop now? Go get 'em girl.

Conclusion

"Now Voyager depart! Much, much for thee is yet in store . . .
now obey, thy cherished, secret wish."
—WALT WHITMAN

Sometimes it takes an extreme for us to make changes in our lives that we should have made years ago. If breast cancer is that extreme for you, then that is the ultimate in making the best of an unfortunate circumstance. If you don't quite feel that way yet, hopefully now that you have read this book you at least no longer look at life as something you once had before cancer. Hopefully you now see life as a beautiful array of possibilities. Your greatest fears were realized when you heard you were diagnosed, but now that you have overcome your disease, it's time to acknowledge that you are a strong, resilient, wise woman who is capable of anything, including joy and pleasure.

Since childhood, you have probably been taught to learn from all of your experiences. If you are lucky and smart, you will take what you learned from your battle with breast cancer and from this book, and apply it to your new life. You will no longer waste your time fretting about things that don't matter. You will no longer hide out at home—you will go outside and embrace all the beauty and love that life has to offer. And you will conquer the sexual fears and unknowns your new body has brought with it.

Acknowledge and appreciate your body as the truly remarkable work of art that it is. Take care of it. Nourish it with only good foods.

Exercise it so it is strong and beautiful. And spend some extra time making yourself up and getting dressed each morning so your inner light can shine through. Eventually, if you follow the advice found within these pages, you will be so far removed from that frightened cancer patient that the real, wonderful you will finally emerge—and you will be better than ever.

This journey to the new you starts emotionally. You must first come to terms with what the onslaught of chemicals, surgeries, and radiation has done to your body and your spirit before you can learn how to heal. You have physical, emotional, and spiritual wounds. Given time, you will discover which are permanent and which are transient. Be patient and kind to yourself, but never settle for the status quo. If you don't like something about your body and it's within your power to change it, do it as soon as possible. If you need help working through certain issues, seek out a counselor or therapist. If the people in your life are toxic, free yourself of them. Never settle for less than anything but love—love for yourself and for those around you.

There is no reason why you cannot have a future filled with happiness. The only thing that can stop you from that is you. However, by taking the initiative to read this book, it means that you see your worth. It means that you want to live, *really* live the rest of your life to the fullest. It is time to once again open yourself up to joy and love, and to reclaim your sexual being. When you do, you will once again be living your life and moving yourself as far away from cancer as you can get. And that, of course, is the best place to be. If you have to push the envelope, step outside your comfort zone, and cross boundaries you never thought you would, so be it. Do whatever is necessary to find your happiness.

Just like your cancer treatments, no one will do this for you. You have to do this on your own, for yourself. When all is said and done and you have once again embraced life and love, the scoreboard will read:

YOU: 1   CANCER: 0

The best is yet to come . . .

$\mathcal{T}$he No Surrender
Breast Cancer
Foundation

The No Surrender Breast Cancer Foundation provides a life-line to women who have just left their doctors' offices after hearing the words, "You have breast cancer." Rather than frantically searching the web for outdated survival statistics, our foundation's comprehensive website offers solid, easy-to-understand information that is specifically written from a patient's point of view.

We take off the "white-coats" and break down the medical lingo that is very hard to decipher under normal circumstances, and impossible under stressful conditions such as a new diagnosis. Piece by piece, we demystify breast cancer and because of the knowledge each woman gains, fear is replaced by empowerment. Through medically sound, doctor reviewed information, everything is explained: Pathology, treatment, types of breasts cancer, surgical options, chemotherapy facts, wigs, nutrition, financial aid, legal resources, the very latest study results, and how to live the best life possible after breast cancer.

The No Surrender Breast Cancer foundation also provides a 24/7, live, peer-driven support forum for women to join and share with other survivors. Here, newly-diagnosed women, seasoned veterans, and advanced-stage women share personal experiences, tips, recommendations, and a deep bond that only survivors can form. It becomes a place where they feel safe to discuss all their fears because they know that their "sisters" will understand them. Oftentimes, as much as they may try, family members really do not comprehend what a woman with breast cancer is truly enduring, which leads to isolation. When she visits the support forum, however, she finds she is no longer alone and gains strength through the other women who are there by her side, fighting with her.

Beyond our foundation's website and support forum, our goal is to save lives. Our "Before Forty Initiative" educates young women about their risks of cancer, particularly triple-negative breast cancer, which appears at an earlier age in women of all races, particularly African American and Hispanic women and in those who carry the BRCA gene. Without swift diagnosis and early, aggressive treatment, triple-negative breast cancer is much harder to fight. Our mission with the Before Forty Initiative is to make the age of baseline diagnostic screenings thirty-five, and the age of screenings for women of high risk, thirty. This includes all methods of screening techniques, including mammography, ultrasound, and breast MRIs. We believe in diligent follow-ups for anything that may be found, and we educate all women that a "watch and wait" strategy is not an option. We are pursuing changing the current guidelines for breast screening and are working towards ensuring coverage for these screenings until "Before Forty" is the standard of care for every woman.

The No Surrender Breast Cancer Foundation is working hard to help women through their cancer and beyond. Women need to become their own advocates and fight for the very best of care; we show them how. We believe that a cure is possible in our lifetime, and we support research towards finding that cure through our No Surrender Breast Cancer Foundation Research Grant program.

"Hope happens here" is not just our motto, but it is our mission: To provide real hope no matter where a woman is in her journey, through education, emotional support, and empowerment.

For more information about the No Surrender
Breast Cancer Foundation, please visit our website at:
www.nosurrenderbreastcancerfoundation.org.

The No Surrender Breast Cancer Foundation is a 501(c) 3, not-for-profit organization.

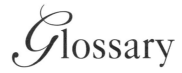

Glossary

adjuvant therapy. Chemotherapy administered after the removal of cancerous tissue to eradicate any underlying, errant cancer cells.

AlloDerm. Tissue matrix from a donor that is added surgically in order to support breast implant reconstruction.

alpha hydroxy acids (AHAs). Ingredient used in chemical peels for faces and in skin treatment products, like moisturizers and cleansers.

anorgasmia. Inability to achieve orgasm.

antioxidants. Vitamins that, when used in cosmetics, act as anti-aging agents and protect against free radicals.

aspirate. To remove fluid and cells from a suspicious area using a small needle.

autologous. Using one's own tissue; an autologous reconstruction uses the patient's own tissue to reconstruct the breast.

axillary. Located under the arm; this area holds the sac of lymph nodes that are first affected by cancer cells.

baseline. A diagnostic test that is done at an early age, before any evidence of disease. It can be used to measure changes in the future and it is recommended when therapy is completed.

benign. Tissue that is not cancerous.

beta hydroxy acids (BHA). Help exfoliate dead skin and clear acne.

bilateral mastectomy. The removal of both breasts.

biopsy. A procedure used on a portion of tissue to determine if it is cancerous.

biotin. A member of the B-complex vitamin that helps hair and nails grow through the formation of glycogen.

botanical. Botanical products are those that are made from plants.

Botox. Injectable, non-toxic form of botulinum toxin A that paralyzes muscles, reducing and/or temporarily eliminating wrinkles on the face and neck.

BRCA1 and BRCA2. The genetic mutation found in heredity breast and ovarian cancer.

bronzers. Cosmetic products that create the illusion of a suntan.

capsular contracture. The formation of scar tissue around a breast implant that tightens the surgical pocket where the implant is placed; it eventually leads to pain and the shifting of implant appearance, and can only be resolved through a surgical procedure to remove the scar tissue.

ceramides. Used in cosmetic products to retain moisture when applied.

cervix. The lower part of the uterus that connects to the vagina.

chemical peel. Chemical solution that improves the skin's appearance.

chemotherapy. A medication designed to target and kill cancer cells throughout the body.

citric acid. Natural astringent and antioxidant.

clear margins. The portion of tissue that surrounds a tumor field that is not affected by cancer; also known as negative margins.

clinical trial. Large-scale research conducted within a controlled group to test, understand, and develop new therapies.

collagen. Found in the human body; as we age it decreases, causing wrinkles. Synthetic forms can be used as cosmetic fillers for wrinkle treatment.

collagen/fat injectable fillers. Fills in wrinkles and fine lines with injectable chemical.

copper peptide. Ingredient in skincare products that soothes and calms the skin.

core needle biopsy. The removal of suspect tissue with a large, hollow needle.

cyst. A fluid-filled lump.

DCIS. Ductal Carcinoma In Situ Cancer that has remained inside the milk duct; considered early-stage cancer.

deep inferior epigastric perforator (DIEP) flap. Reconstruction technique that uses fat and tissue from the abdomen and, through microsurgical techniques, transfers blood vessels to the chest and connects them to the existing blood supply to create a new breast.

dermabrasion. The removal of dead skin and fine wrinkles through the use of chemical and/or abrasive agents.

distant recurrence. A return of breast cancer to a location other than the breast area. For instance, it may recur in the lung, bone, brain, liver, etc.

drain. A plastic tube with a bulbous container at one end that drains the excess fluid from a post-surgical site, such as the underarm. The tube is inserted during surgery through a tiny opening in the skin.

dyspareunia. Pain some women experience during sexual intercourse.

elastin. Elastin is used in cosmetics to protect the skin from getting dry.

ER+. Cancer that has estrogen receptors and needs estrogen to grow.

ER-. Cancer that does not have estrogen receptors and is not affected by estrogen.

estrogen. A female hormone.

evening primrose oil; gamma linolenic acid (GLA). Can be used topically as a facial moisturizer, and can also be used to increase moisture in the vaginal tissues.

excisional biopsy. A procedure that is done to remove a suspicious area or lump, as well as the margins that surround it.

expander. Balloon-shaped device used to open the pocket under the pectoral muscle in order to create space for the placement of a breast implant.

female hypoactive sexual desire (HSDD). Loss of libido in women.

flap surgery. Surgery that involves the use of tissue from one of a number of locations of the body to create a breast .

forehead lift. Surgically removing excess fat and skin, followed by pulling the muscles to open the eyes and reduce heavy brows.

gluteal artery perforator (GAP) flap. Reconstructive technique that uses tissue from the buttocks and transfers the blood supply to the chest to form a breast.

glycerin. Used in cosmetic products to hold moisture against the skin and prevent dryness.

glycolic acid (hydroxyacetic acid). Used to exfoliate skin in low concentrations, or as a chemical peel in larger concentrations.

hormone receptor. Cells that are fed by hormones and can be treated with hormonal therapy.

hormone therapy. Orally, estrogen can be taken to reduce the effects of menopause; topically, it can be used to return lubrication to vaginal tissues.

hyaluronic acid. Part of human connective tissue; it has been synthesized into skincare products to increase moisture and decrease wrinkles and the signs of aging.

hydrolyzed ascorbic acid. Antioxidant skincare product that stimulates the growth of collagen.

hydroquinone. A chemical found in products used to lighten the skin.

hydroxy acids. Used in skincare products to reduce wrinkles and sagging; can reverse the signs of aging.

in situ. A growth or grouping of cells that remains in place within the ducts or lobules.

incisional biopsy. A procedure that is done to remove a portion of tissue from a large lump or suspicious area, while leaving the remaining lump or area in tact.

invasive. Cancer that has grown outside of the point of origin, or that has broken free of the ducts or lobules.

Juvaderm. Injectable filler that smoothes facial lines and wrinkles.

latissimus dorsi flap (LD flap). A breast reconstruction surgery that uses the latissimus dorsi muscle to recreate a breast mound.

LCIS. Lobular cancer in situ; an area of pre-cancerous tissue that remains inside the milk lobule.

libido. Sex drive.

local recurrence. A return of cancer to the point of origin, such as the scar line or another part of the same breast.

lubricant (lube). A thick liquid or gel that makes sexual intercourse more enjoyable by easing dryness problems and pain.

lumpectomy. A procedure that is done to remove a cancerous area or tumor, as well as the surrounding margins.

lymph nodes. Glands that filter impurities throughout the body.

lymphatic system. Circulatory system that consists of the nodes, lymphatic fluid, and blood supply.

malignant. A tissue or lump that has been found to have cancer cells.

mastectomy. Surgical removal of a breast, usually to remove cancerous tissue.

metastasis. The spread of cancer to either a local area near the breast, or to distant organs or bones.

negative lymph nodes. Lymph nodes that are clear of cancer cells; also known as node negative.

neo adjuvant therapy. The administration of chemotherapeutic agents to shrink the cancerous area before surgical removal.

oncologist. The doctor who specializes in the study of blood and the administration of chemotherapeutic agents.

oophrectomy. The surgical removal of ovaries.

palpable. Can be felt by hand.

para-aminobenzoic acid (PABA). B-complex vitamin that is used in sunscreen.

pathologist. A doctor who examines cells to determine if they are cancerous.

pathology laboratory. Where pathologists work.

pathology report. A compilation of the pathologists findings.

photoaging. The effect of the sun's damage on the skin.

phytocosmetics. Cosmetic products that are made with natural ingredients from plants.

positive lymph nodes. Lymph nodes that have cancer cells in them; also known as node positive.

positive margin. The tissue surrounding a cancerous area or tumor that also contains cancer cells.

PR+. Cancer that has progesterone receptors and needs progesterone to grow.

PR-. Cancer that does not have progesterone receptors and is not affected by progesterone.

progesterone. A female hormone.

prognosis. An educated guess or prediction of a patient's outcome.

prophylactic mastectomy. The removal of one or both breasts in order to prevent or reduce the risk of cancer occurring in them.

radiation oncologist. The doctor who specializes in radiation and the administration of radiotherapy.

Radiesse. Injectable filler that smooths out facial wrinkles.

reconstructive plastic surgery. The recreation of a breast in women who have had a mastectomy; there are many different techniques ranging from implants to microsurgery.

Restylane. Dermal filler used to smooth out wrinkles.

Retinol (vitamin A). Main ingredient in Retin A; reduces wrinkles and smoothes skin by increasing collagen.

salicylic acid. Used in cosmetic treatments to remove dead layers of skin, revealing fresher, clearer skin underneath.

sentinel node biopsy. The identification and removal of the first-in-line lymph node (sentinel) that would be affected by a spread of cancer cells to the lymphatic system.

stereotactic biopsy. A needle biopsy guided by either ultrasound or mammogram.

subcutaneous mastectomy. A procedure that removes all breast tissue but preserves the breast skin and nipple; also known as the skin-sparing procedure.

tartaric acid. Tartaric acid comes from apples and is used to promote the texture and tone of the skin.

tissue expansion. A surgical procedure that involves inserting a balloon-like device (called an expander) under the skin. The expander is then slowly filled to stretch and expand the skin in order to make room for an implant to be placed.

tocopherol (vitamin E). Helps the skin reproduce healthy new tissue.

transverse rectus abdominis myocutaneous (TRAM) flap. A breast reconstruction technique that utilizes the abdominal muscles and blood supply to create a new breast.

transverse upper gracilis (TUG) flap. Transfering thigh tissue and the gracilis muscle to create a new breast using microsurgical technique.

Tretinoin. The acid form of vitamin A; it reduces wrinkles and smoothes skin by increasing collagen.

ubiquinone idebenone. Powerful antioxidants that aid in reducing wrinkles.

ultrasound (sonogram). Device that utilizes sound waves to create images of tissue.

vaginal dialators. Graduated, small devices that are used to open the muscles of the vagina and reverse atrophy.

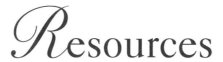

Resources

There is help available to you if you know where to look. This guide offers suggested resources, products, and organizations. Whether you are looking for personal counseling or personal lubricant, the following information should help you on your way.

COUNSELORS, THERAPISTS, AND PSYCHIATRISTS

If you are looking for general psychological assistance or for a marriage counselor in your area, these organizations can help direct you to local resources.

American Psychotherapy Association
http://www.americanpsychotherapy.com/services/therapist/

Family and Marriage Counseling
http://family-marriage-counseling.com

The National Registry of Family and Marriage Counseling
http://www.counsel-search.com

SEX THERAPY RESOURCES

If you are looking for counselors or doctors who can help you with more intimate issues, these organizations will help you find someone near you.

American Association of Sex Educators, Counselors, and Therapists (AASECT)
http://www.aasect.org

American College of Obstetricians and Gynecologists (ACOG)
http://www.acog.org

American Social Health Association (ASHA)
http://www.ashastd.org

International Academy of Sex Research (IASR)
http://www.iasr.org

International Association for the Treatment of Sexual Offenders (IATSO)
http://www.medacad.org/iatso/

International Society for the Study of Women's Sexual Health (ISSWSH)
http://www.isswsh.org

Kinsey Institute for Research in Sex, Gender, and Reproduction
http://www.indiana.edu/~kinsey/

National Vulvodynia Association (NVA)
http://www.nva.org

National Women's Health Network
http://www.womenshealthnetwork.org

North American Menopause Society (NAMS)
http://www.menopause.org

Planned Parenthood
http://www.plannedparenthood.org

Sexuality Information and Education Council of the U.S. (SIECUS)
http://www.siecus.org

Society for the Scientific Study of Sexuality (SSSS)
http://www.sexscience.org

Society for Women's Health Research
http://www.womenshealthresearch.org

World Association for Sexual Health
http://www.worldsexualhealth.com

LEGAL RESOURCES

If you are looking for legal assistance with adoption or to find out what your options are if you are considering divorce, please contact one of the following organizations.

Adoption Information
http://www.adopting.org

Adoption Information through the Government
http://www.childwelfare.gov

Adoption Resources
http://www.adoption.com

Divorce Law Resource
http://www.divorcelawinfo.com

Divorce Support
http://www.divorcesupport.com

International Adoption Resources
http://internationaladoptionre-sources.org

POST-SURGICAL AND RECONSTRUCTION RESOURCES

These organizations offer information on plastic and reconstructive surgery, lymphedema support, and care and support for women who choose not to reconstruct.

American Society of Plastic Surgeons
www.plasticsurgery.org

Breast Free - Choosing to live life without Reconstruction
www.breastfree.org

Breast Reconstruction.org - Comprehensive resource for Breast Reconstruction
www.breastreconstruction.org

Breastimplantsafety.org
www.breastimplantsafety.org

The Breast Reconstruction Guidebook
www.breastrecon.com

Image Reborn
www.imagerebornfoundation.org

Lymphedema Support and Resources - Step Up - Speak Out
www.stepupspeakout.org

My Hope Chest
www.myhopechest.org

National Lymphedema Network
www.lymphnet.org

Shop Well With You
www.shopwellwithyou.org

Staying Abreast
www.stayingabreast.com

SEXUAL AIDS

If visiting an adult store is not for you, these resources offer a discreet online shopping experience.

Adam and Eve
http://www.adamandevetoys.com

Babeland
http://www.babeland.com

Drug Store
http://www.drugstore.com

Eve's Garden
http://www.evesgarden.com

Good Vibrations
http://www.goodvibes.com

The Magic Wand Shop
http://www.hitachi-magic-wand.com

Ohmybod - The Ipod Vibrator
http://www.ohmibod.com

Spicy Gear
http://www.spicygear.com

LUBRICATION AND AROUSAL PRODUCTS

Here is a guide to the most popular products to enhance and help your sexual experience.

AstroGlide
www.astroglide.com

Pjur Brand
www.pjur.com

Emerita Brands
www.emerita.com

Replens
www.replens.com

KY Brands
www.k-y.com

Zestra
www.zestra.com

WEBISTES WITH RESEARCH INFORMATION

These online resources provide extensive information about breast cancer. Many also offer online support communities.

No Surrender Breast Cancer Foundation
www.nosurrenderbreastcancerfoundation.org

American Cancer Society
www.acs.org

American Society of Clinical Oncology
www.www.asco.org

Breast Cancer Organization
http://www.breastcancer.org

Breast Free
www.breastfree.org

Breast Reconstruction
www.breastreconstruction.org

Facing Our Risk of Cancer Empowered (Genetic Breast Cancer)
www.facingourrisk.org

Fertile Hope
www.fertilehope.org

Imaginis
www.imaginis.com

Journal of Clinical Oncology
www.jco.org

Lance Armstrong Foundation
www.laf.org

Lymphedema Support by Survivors
stepupspeakout.org

National Lymphedema Network
www.lymphnet.org

Planet Cancer
www.planetcancer.org

SHARE: Self-help for Women with Breast or Ovarian Cancer
www.sharecancersupport.org

The Susan G. Komen Breast Cancer Foundation, Inc.
www.komen.org

Young Survival Coalition
www.youngsurvival.org

References

Chapter 1

Abraham, J., Haut, M.W., Moran, M.T., Filburn, S., Iannetti, M.P., Lemiuex, S., Kuwabara, H. "The effect of chemotherapy for breast cancer on cerebral white matter: A diffusion tensor imaging study." *Am Soc Clin Oncol.* 2005; Abstract No: 606.

Bar Ad, V., Cheville, A., Amin, N., Booty, J., Solin, L.J., Harris, E.E. "Minimal arm lymphedema after breast conservation therapy." *Journ Clin Oncol.* 2006; ASCO Annual Meeting Proceedings Part I. Vol 24, No. 18S. Abstract No: 10527.

Donovan, K.A., Jacobsen, P.B., Andrykowski, M.A., et al. "Course of fatigue in women receiving chemotherapy and/or radiotherapy for early stage breast cancer." *J Pain Symptom Manage.* 2004; 28: 373-380.

Early Breast Cancer Trialists' Collaboration Group (EBCTCG). "Effects of chemotherapy and hormonal therapy for early breast cancer on recurrence and 15-year survival: An overview of the randomised trials." *Lancet.* 2005.

Hafner, A., Robinson, R., Massa, L., Maddox, J., Hoskins, C., Morgan, S., Reid, T. "Combined Modality Treatment of Lymphedema using the Reid Sleeve and the BioCompression/Optiflow System." *Am Soc Clin Oncol.* 2005; Abstract No: 592.

Kim, S. H., Park, B.W., Ahn, S. H., Noh, D.Y., Nam, S. J., Lee, E.S., Yun, Y.H. "Prevalence and correlates of fatigue and depression in breast cancer survivors: Breast cancer quality care study." *J Clin Oncol.* 2006; ASCO Annual Meeting Proceedings Part I. Vol 24, No 18S Abstract No: 683.

Lopez, A., Avery, D.J., Hofacre, M.B. "Assessing the Needs of Long-term Breast Cancer Survivors." *Am Soc Clin Oncol.* 2005; Abstract No: 817.

Mathew, J., Barthelmes, L., Neminathan, S., Crawford, D., Ysbyty, G. "Comparative study of lymphedema with axillary node dissection and axillary sampling with radiotherapy in women undergoing breast conservation surgery for breast cancer." *San Antonio Breast Cancer Symposium.* Dec 2005; 1003.

Naughton, M. J., Petrek, J. A., Ip, E., Paskett, E. D., Naftalis, E. "Health-Related Quality of Life of Pre-Menopausal Breast Cancer Survivors." *Am Soc Clin Oncol.* 2005; Abstract No: 636

Servaes, P., Verhagen, S., Bleijenberg, G. "Determinants of chronic fatigue in disease-free breast cancer patients: A cross-sectional study." *Ann Oncol.* 2002; 13: 589-598.

Visovsky, C., Collins, M., Abbott, L., Aschenbrenner, J., Hart, C. "Putting evidence into practice: Evidence-based interventions for chemotherapy-induced peripheral neuropathy." *Clin J Oncol Nurs.* 2007; 11: 901-913.

Wickham, R. "Chemotherapy-induced peripheral neuropathy: A review and implications for oncology nursing practice." *Clin J Oncol Nurs.* 2007; 11.

Chapter 2

Early Breast Cancer Trialists' Collaboration Group (EBCTCG). "Effects of chemotherapy and hormonal therapy for early breast cancer on recurrence and 15-year survival: An overview of the randomised trials." *Lancet.* 2005.

Kim, S. H., Park, B.W., Ahn, S. H., Noh, D.Y., Nam, S. J., Lee, E.S., Yun, Y.H. "Prevalence and correlates of fatigue and depression in breast cancer survivors: Breast cancer quality care study." *J Clin Oncol.* 2006; ASCO Annual Meeting Proceedings Part I Vol 24, No 18S, Abstract No: 683.

Loftus, L.S., Laronga, C. "Evaluating Patients With Chronic Pain After Breast Cancer Surgery: The Search for Relief." *JAMA.* 2009.

Chapter 3

Abrahamson, P.E., Gammon, M.D., Lund, M.J., Britton, J.A., Marshall, S.W., Flagg, E.W., et al. "Recreational physical activity and survival among young women with breast cancer." *Cancer.* 2006.

Berstad, P., Ma, H., Bernstein, L., Ursin, G. "Alcohol intake and breast cancer risk among young women." *Breast Cancer Res Treat.* 2008.

Bessaoud, F., Daurès, J.P. "Patterns of Alcohol (Especially Wine) Consumption and Breast Cancer Risk: A Case-Control Study among a Population in Southern France." *Ann Epidemiol.* 2008; Apr 25.

Byers, T., Nestle, M., McTiernan, A., et al. "American cancer society guidelines on nutrition and physical activity for cancer prevention: reducing the risk of cancer with healthy food choices and physical activity." *CA Cancer J Clin*. 2002.

Cade J.E., Burley, V.J., Greenwood, D.C. "Dietary fibre and risk of breast cancer in the UK Women's Cohort Study." *Int J Epidemiol*. 2007.

Campbell, K.L., Westerlind, K.C., Harber, V.J., Bell, G.J., Mackey, J.R., Courneya, K.S. "Effects of aerobic exercise training on estrogen metabolism in premenopausal women: a randomized controlled trial." *Cancer Epidemiol Biomarkers Prev*. 2007.

Chen, W.Y., Willett, W.C., Rosner, B., Colditz, G.A. "Moderate alcohol consumption and breast cancer risk." *ASCO Annual Meeting*. 2005; Abstract 515.

Chlebowski, R.T., Blackburn, G.L., Elashoff, R.E., Thomson, C., Goodman, M.T., Shapiro, A., Giuliano, A.E., Karanja, N., Hoy, M.K., Nixon, D.W. "The WINS Investigators Dietary fat reduction in postmenopausal women with primary breast cancer: Phase III Women's Intervention Nutrition Study (WINS)." *Am Soc Clin Oncol*. 2005; Abstract No: 10.

Chlebowski, R.T., Blackburn, G.I., Thomson, C.A., et al. "Dietary fat reduction and breast cancer outcome: Interim efficacy results from the Women's Intervention Nutrition Study." *Journal of the National Cancer Institute*. 2006.

Cramp, F., Daniel, J. "Exercise for the management of cancer-related fatigue in adults." *Cochrane Database Syst Rev*. 2008.

Daley, A.J., Crank, H., Saxton, J.M., Mutrie, N., Coleman, R., Roalfe, A. "Randomized trial of exercise therapy in women treated for breast cancer." *J Clin Oncol*. 2007.

de Lima, F.E., do Rosário Dias de Oliveira Latorre, M., de Carvalho Costa, M.J., Fisberg, R.M. "Diet and cancer in Northeast Brazil: evaluation of eating habits and food group consumption in relation to breast cancer." *Cad Saude Publica*. 2008.

Freiman, A., Bird, G., Metelitsa, A.I., Barankin, B., Cutaneous, G.J.L. "Effects of Smoking." *Journal of Cutaneous Medicine and Surgery: Incorporating Medical and Surgical Dermatology*. 2004; Vol 8, No 6.

Garland, C.F., Garland, F.C., Gorham, E.D., et al. "The role of vitamin D in cancer prevention." *American Journal of Public Health*. 2006.

Gaudet, M.M., Britton, J.A., Kabat, G.C., Steck-Scott, S., Eng, S.M., Teitelbaum, S.L., et al. "Fruits, vegetables, and micronutrients in relation to breast cancer modified by menopause and hormone receptor status." *Cancer Epidemiol Biomarkers Prev.* 2004.

Heaney, R.P. "Vitamin D in health and disease." *Clinical Journal of the American Society of Nephrology.* 2008.

Hirose, K., Matsuo, K., Iwata, H., Tajima, K. "Dietary patterns and the risk of breast cancer in Japanese women." *Cancer Science.* 2007.

Holick, C.N., Newcomb, P.A., Trentham-Dietz, A., Titus-Ernstoff, L., Bersch, A.J., Stampfer, M.J., et al. "Physical activity and survival after diagnosis of invasive breast cancer." *Cancer Epidemiol Biomarkers Prev.* 2008.

Holick, M.F. "Vitamin D deficiency." *New England Journal of Medicine.* 2007.

Holmes, M.D., Chen, W.Y., Feskanich, D., Kroenke, C.H., Colditz, G.A. "Physical activity and survival after breast cancer diagnosis." *JAMA.* 2005.

Irwin, M.L., Aiello, E.J., McTiernan, A., Bernstein, L., Gilliland, F.D., Baumgartner, R.N., et al. "Physical activity, body mass index, and mammographic density in postmenopausal breast cancer survivors." *J Clin Oncol.* 2007.

Iwasaki, M., Otani, T., Inoue, M., Sasazuki, S., Tsugane, S. "Body size and risk for breast cancer in relation to estrogen and progesterone receptor status in Japan." *Ann Epidemiol.* 2007.

Kim, E.H., Willett, W.C., Colditz, G.A., et al. "Dietary fat and risk of postmenopausal breast cancer in a 20-year follow-up." *American Journal of Epidemiology.* 2006.

Kroenke, C.H., Chen, W.Y., Rosner, B., Holmes, M.D. "Weight, weight gain, and survival after breast cancer diagnosis." *J Clin Oncol.* 2005.

Kushi, L.H., Byers, T., Doyle, C., et al. "American Cancer Society Guidelines on Nutrition and Physical Activity for cancer prevention: Reducing the risk of cancer with healthy food choices and physical activity." *CA Cancer J Clin.* 2006.

Lahmann, P.H., Friedenreich, C., Schuit, A.J., Salvini, S., Allen, N.E., Key, T.J., et al. "Physical activity and breast cancer risk: the European Prospective Investigation into Cancer and Nutrition." *Cancer Epidemiol Biomarkers Prev.* 2007.

Lappe, J.M., Travers-Gustafson, D., Davies, K.M., Recker, R.R., Heaney, R.P. "Vitamin D and calcium supplementation reduces cancer risk: Results of a randomized trial." *American Journal of Clinical Nutrition.* 2007.

Ligibel, J.A., Campbell, N., Partridge, A., Chen, W.Y., Salinardi, T., Chen, H., et al. "Impact of a mixed strength and endurance exercise intervention on insulin levels in breast cancer survivors." *J Clin Oncol.* 2008.

Lissowska, J., Gaudet, M.M., Brinton, L.A., Peplonska, B., Sherman, M., Szeszenia-Dabrowska, N., et al. "Intake of fruits, and vegetables in relation to breast cancer risk by hormone receptor status." *Breast Cancer Res Treat.* 2008.

Loi, S., Milne, R.L., Friedlander, M.L., McCredie, M.R., Giles, G.G., Hopper, J.L., et al. "Obesity and outcomes in premenopausal and postmenopausal breast cancer." *Cancer Epidemiol Biomarkers Prev.* 2005.

McCarty, M.F. "A low-fat, whole-food vegan diet, as well as other strategies that down-regulate IGF-I activity, may slow the human aging process." *Med. Hypotheses.* 2003.

McEligot, A.J., Largent, J., Ziogas, A., Peel, D., Anton-Culver, H. "Dietary fat, fiber, vegetable, and micronutrients are associated with overall survival in post menopausal women diagnosed with breast cancer." *Nutr Cancer.* 2006.

Melamed, M.L., Michos, E.D., Post, W., Astor, B. "25-hydroxyvitamin D levels and the risk of mortality in the general population." *Archives of Internal Medicine.* 2008.

Monninkhof, E.M., Elias, S.G., Vlems, F.A., van der Tweel, I., Schuit, A.J., Voskuil, D.W., et al. "Physical activity and breast cancer: a systematic review." *Epidemiology.* 2007.

Pierce, J.P., Natarajan, L., Caan, B.J., Parker, B.A., Greenberg, E.R., Flatt, S.W., et al. "Influence of a diet very high in vegetables, fruit, and fiber and low in fat on prognosis following treatment for breast cancer: the Women's Healthy Eating and Living (WHEL) randomized trial." *JAMA.* 2007.

Pierce J.P., Stefanick, M.L., Flatt, S.W., et al. "Greater survival after breast cancer in physically active women with high vegetable-fruit intake regardless of obesity." *J Clin Oncol.* 2007.

Prentice, R.L., Caan, B., Chlebowski, R.T., et al. "Low-fat dietary pattern and risk of invasive breast cancer: The Women's Health Initiative Randomized Controlled Dietary Modification Trial." *Journal of the American Medical Association.* 2006.

Reeves, G.K., Pirie, K., Beral, V., Green, J., Spencer, E., Bull, D. "Million Women Study Collaboration. Cancer incidence and mortality in relation to body mass index in the Million Women Study: cohort study." *BMJ.* 2007.

Riboli, E., Norat, T. "Epidemiologic evidence of the protective effect of fruit and vegetables on cancer risk." *Am J Clin Nutr.* 2003.

Rock, C.L., Flatt, S.W., Natarajan, L., Thomson, C.A., Bardwell, W.A., Newman, V.A., et al. "Plasma carotenoids and recurrence-free survival in women with a history of breast cancer." *J Clin Oncol.* 2005.

Rock, C.L., Flatt, S.W., Thomson, C.A., Stefanick, M.L., Newman, V.A., Jones, L.A., et al. "Effects of a high-fiber, low-fat diet intervention on serum concentrations of reproductive steroid hormones in women with a history of breast cancer." *J Clin Oncol.* 2004.

Sant, M., Allemani, C., Sieri, S., Krogh, V., Menard, S., Tagliabue, E., et al. "Salad vegetables dietary pattern protects against HER-2- positive breast cancer: a prospective Italian study." *Int J Cancer.* 2007.

Schulz, M., Hoffmann, K., Weikert, C., Nöthlings, U., Schulze, M.B., Boeing, H. "Identification of a dietary pattern characterized by high-fat food choices associated with increased risk of breast cancer: the European Prospective Investigation into Cancer and Nutrition (EPIC)-Potsdam Study." *Br J Nutr.* 2008.

Slavin, J.L. "Mechanisms for the impact of whole grain foods on cancer risk." *J Am Coll Nutr.* 2000.

Suzuki, R., Orsini, N., Mignone, L., Saji, S., Wolk, A. "Alcohol intake and risk of breast cancer defined by estrogen and progesterone receptor status—a meta-analysis of epidemiological studies." *Int J Cancer.* 2008.

Suzuki, R., Ye, W., Rylander-Rudqvist, T., Saji, S., Colditz, G.A., Wolk, A. "Alcohol and postmenopausal breast cancer risk defined by estrogen and progesterone receptor status: a prospective cohort study." *J Natl Cancer.*

Tavani, A., Giordano, L., Gallus, S., Talamini, R., Franceschi, S., Giacosa, A., et al. "Consumption of sweet foods and breast cancer risk in Italy." *Ann Oncol.* 2006.

Tjonneland, A., Christensen, J., Thomsen, B.L., Olsen, A., Stripp, C., Overvad, K., et al. "Lifetime alcohol consumption and postmenopausal breast cancer rate in Denmark: a prospective cohort study." *J Nutr.* 2004.

Travis, R.C., Allen, N.E., Appleby, P.N., Spencer, E.A., Roddam, A.W., Key, T.J. "A prospective study of vegetarianism and isoflavone intake in relation to breast cancer risk in British women." *Int J Cancer.* 2008.

Valenti, M., Porzio, G., Aielli, F., Verna, L., Cannita, K., Manno, R., Masedu, F., Marchetti, P., Ficorella, C. "Physical exercise and quality of life in breast cancer survivors." *Int J Med Sci.* 2008.

Visvanathan, K., Crum, R.M., Strickland, P.T., You, X., Ruczinski, I., Berndt, S.I., et al. "Alcohol dehydrogenase genetic polymorphisms, low-to-moderate alcohol consumption, and risk of breast cancer." *Alcohol Clin Exp Res.* 2007.

Whiteman, M.K., Hillis, S.D., Curtis, K.M., McDonald, J.A., Wingo, P.A., Marchbanks, P.A. "Body mass and mortality after breast cancer diagnosis." *Cancer Epidemiol Biomarkers Prev.* 2005.

World Cancer Research Fund. "Food, nutrition, physical activity, and the prevention of cancer: a global perspective." *American Institute for Cancer Research.* 2007.

Yumuk, P.F., Dane, F., Yumuk, V.D., Yazici, D., Ege, B., Bekiroglu, N., et al. "Impact of body mass index on cancer development." *J BUON.* 2008.

Zhang, S.M., Lee, I.M., Manson, J.E., Cook, N.R., Willett, W.C., Buring, J.E. "Alcohol consumption and breast cancer risk in the Women's Health Study." *Am J Epidemiol.* 2007.

Chapter 4

Woodson, S.A. "Latisse: Empirical Discovery Yields Treatment for Sparse Eyelashes." *Nurses Womens Health.* Jun 2009.

Chapter 6

Abraham, J.,. Haut, M.W, Moran, M.T., Filburn, S., Iannetti, M.P., Lemiuex, S., Kuwabara, H. "The effect of chemotherapy for breast cancer on cerebral white matter: A diffusion tensor imaging study." *Am Soc Clin Oncol.* 2005; Abstract No: 606.

Barnes, P.M., Bloom, B., Nahin, R. "Complementary and alternative medicine use among adults and children: United States, 2007." *CDC National Health Statistics Report 12.* 2008.

Bremer, E., Samplonius, D.F., van Genne, lL., Dijkstra, M.H., Kroesen, B.J., de Leij L.F.M.H., Helfrich, W. "Simultaneous Inhibition of Epidermal Growth Factor Receptor (EGFR) Signaling and Enhanced Activation of Tumor Necrosis Factor-related Apoptosis-inducing Ligand (TRAIL) Receptor-mediated Apoptosis Induction by an scFv:sTRAIL Fusion Protein with Specificity for Human EGFR." *J. Biol. Chem.* 2005; Mar 18.

Broekel, J.A., Thors, C.L., Jacobsen, P.B., Small, M., Cox, C.E. "Sexual functioning in long-term breast cancer survivors treated with adjuvant chemotherapy." *Breast Cancer Research Treatment.* 2002.

Brown, B.D., Thomas, W., Hutchins, A., Martini, M.C., Slavin, J.L. "Types of dietary fat and soy minimally affect hormones and biomarkers associated with breast cancer risk in premenopausal women." *Nutr Cancer.* 2002.

Brown, J.S., Vittinghoff, E., Kanaya, A.M., et al. "Urinary tract infections in postmenopausal women: Effect of hormone therapy and risk factors." *Obstet Gynecol.* 2001.

Bruno, D., Feeney, K.J. "Management of postmenopausal symptoms in breast cancer survivors." *Semin Oncol.* 2006.

Carroll, D.G. "Nonhormonal therapies for hot flashes in menopause." *Am Fam Physician.* 2006.

Castelo-Branco, C., Cancelo, M.J., Villero, J., et al. "Management of post-menopausal vaginal atrophy and atrophic vaginitis." *Maturitas.* 2005; 52 (suppl 1).

Chen, J., Stavro, P.M., Thompson, L.U. "Dietary flaxseed inhibits human breast cancer growth and metastasis and downregulates expression of insulin-like growth factor and epidermal growth factor receptor." *Nutr Cancer.* 2002.

Chen, J., Wang, L., Thompson, L.U. "Flaxseed and its components reduce metastasis after surgical excision of solid human breast tumor in nude mice." *Cancer Lett.* 2005; May 20.

Clemons, M., Simmons, C. "Identifying menopause in breast cancer patients: Considerations and implications." *Breast Cancer Res Treat.* 2007;104:115–120.

Cohen, S.M., O'Connor, A.M., Hart, J., Merel, N.H., Te, H.S. "Autoimmune hepatitis associated with the use of black cohosh: a case study." *Menopause.* 2004;11:575–577.

Cos, S., Martinez-Campa, C., Mediavilla, M.D., Sanchez-Barcelo, E.J. "Melatonin modulates aromatase activity in MCF-7 human breast cancer cells." *J Pineal Res.* 2005.

Davis, V., et al. "Effects of black cohosh on mammary tumor development and progression in MMTV-neu transgenic mice." *Proceedings of the American Association of Cancer Research.* Jul 2003; Abstract No: R1 90, Vol 44, 2nd ed.

del Rio, B., Garcia Pedrero, J.M., Martinez-Campa, C., Zuazua, P., Lazo, P.S., Ramos, S. "Melatonin, an endogenous-specific inhibitor of estrogen receptor alpha via calmodulin." *J Biol Chem.* 2004.

Early Breast Cancer Trialists' Collaboration Group (EBCTCG). "Effects of chemotherapy and hormonal therapy for early breast cancer on recurrence and 15-year survival: An overview of the randomised trials." *Lancet.* 2005.

Fann, J.R., Thomas-Rich, A.M., Katon, W.J., Cowley, D., Pepping, M., McGregor, B.A., Gralow, J. "Major depression after breast cancer: a review of epidemiology and treatment." *Gen Hosp Psychiatry.* 2008.

Ganz, P.A. "Breast cancer, menopause, and long-term survivorship: Critical issues for the 21st century." *Am J Med.* 2005; 118.

Gupta, P., Sturdee, D.W., Palin, S.L., et al. "Menopausal symptoms in women treated for breast cancer: The prevalence and severity of symptoms and their perceived effects on quality of life." *Climacteric.* 2006.

Helferich, W. "Soy May Increase Breast Cancer Growth, American Cancer Society." *Cancer Research.* 2001; Vol 61.

Hill, S.M., Collins, A., Kiefer, T.L. "The modulation of oestrogen receptor-alpha activity by melatonin in MCF-7 human breast cancer cells." *Eur J Cancer.* 2000.

Hu, K.K., Boyko, E.J., Scholes, D., et al. "Risk factors for urinary tract infections in postmenopausal women." *Arch Intern Med.* 2004.

Jin, Y., Desta, Z., Stearns, V., Ward, B., Ho, H., Lee, K.H., Skaar, T., Storniolo, A.M., Li, L., Araba, A., Blanchard, R., Nguyen, A., Ullmer, L., Hayden, J., Lemler, S., Weinshilboum, R.M., Rae, J.M., Hayes, D.F., Flockhart, D.A. "CYP2D6 genotype, antidepressant use, and tamoxifen metabolism during adjuvant breast cancer treatment." *J Natl Cancer Inst.* 2005.

Kendall, A., Dowsett, M., Folkerd, E., et al. "Caution: Vaginal estradiol appears to be contraindicated in postmenopausal women on adjuvant aromatase inhibitors." *Ann Oncol.* 2006.

Key, T., Appleby, P., Barnes, I., et al. "Endogenous Hormones and Breast Cancer Collaborative Group. Endogenous sex hormones and breast cancer in postmenopausal women: Reanalysis of nine prospective studies." *J Natl Cancer Inst.* 2002.

Kim, S.H., Park, B.W., Ahn, S.H., Noh, D.Y., Nam, S.J., Lee, E.S., Yun, Y.H. "Prevalence and correlates of fatigue and depression in breast cancer survivors: Breast cancer quality care study." *J Clin Oncol.* 2006; ASCO Annual Meeting Proceedings Part I, Vol 24, No18S, Abstract No: 683.

Lam, M.S.H., Ignoffo, R.J. "A Guide to Clinically Relevant Drug Interactions in Oncology." *Oncol Pharm Pract.* Jun 1, 2003.

Lin, N.U., Winer, E.P. "Advances in Adjuvant Endocrine Therapy for Post-menopausal Women." *J Clin Oncol.* Feb 2008.

Lopez, A., Avery, D.J., Hofacre, M.B. "Assessing the Needs of Long-term Breast Cancer Survivors." *Am Soc Clin Oncol.* 2005; Abstract No: 817.

Loprinzi, C.L., Sloan, J.A., Stearns, V., Diekmann, B., Novotny, P.J., Kimmick, G., Gordon, P., Pandya, K.J., Guttuso, T., Reddy, S. "Newer antidepressants and gabapentin for hot flashes: an individual subject pooled analysis." *J Clin Oncol.* 2008.

Lynch, C.R., Folkers, M.E., Hutson, W.R. "Fulminant hepatic failure associated with the use of black cohosh: a case report." *Liver Transpl.* 2006.

Mackay, D., Miller, A.L. "Nutritional Support for Wound Healing." *Alternate Medicine Review.* 2003; Vol 8, No 4.

Maroon, J., Bost, J. "Omega 3 Fatty acids (fish oil) as an anti-inflammatory: an alternative to nonsteroidal anti-inflammatory drugs for discogenic pain." *Surgical Neurology.* 2006; Vol 65, Iss 4: 326-331.

Maurer, H.R. "Bromelain: Biochemistry, pharmacology and medical use." *Cellular and Molecular Life Sciences.* Aug 2001;Vol 58, No 9.

Meletis, C.D. "Natural Reief of Sprains, Strains and Arthritis." *Alternative and Complementary Therapies.* Jun 2000.

Morales, L., Neven, P., Timmerman, D., et al. "Acute effects of tamoxifen and third-generation aromatase inhibitors on menopausal symptoms of breast cancer patients." *Anticancer Drugs.* 2004.

Naughton, M.J., Petrek, J.A., Ip, E., Paskett, E.D., Naftalis, E. "Health-Related Quality of Life of Pre-Menopausal Breast Cancer Survivors." *Am Soc Clin Oncol.* 2005; Abstract No: 636.

Nilsson, S., Makela, S., Treuter, E., et al. "Mechanisms of estrogen action." *Physiol Rev.* 2001; 81:1535–1565.

Notelovitz, M., Funk, S., Nanavati, N., et al. "Estradiol absorption from vaginal tablets in postmenopausal women." *Obstet Gynecol.* 2002.

Pritchard, K.I., Khan, H., Levine, M. "Clinical practice guidelines for the care and treatment of breast cancer: 14. The role of hormone replacement therapy in women with a previous diagnosis of breast cancer." *CMAJ.* 2002.

Radimer, K., Bindewald, B., Hughes, J., et al. "Dietary supplement use by US adults: data from the National Health and Nutrition Examination Survey, 1999–2000." *American Journal of Epidemiology.* 2004.

Rioux, J.E., Devlin, C., Gelfand, M.M., et al. "17 -estradiol vaginal tablet versus conjugated equine estrogen vaginal cream to relieve menopausal atrophic vaginitis." *Menopause.* 2000.

Rockwell, S., Liu, Y., Higgins, S.A. "Alteration of the effects of cancer therapy agents on breast cancer cells by the herbal medicine black cohosh." *Breast Cancer Res Treat.* 2005.

Rockwell, S. Yale Cancer Center, Yale Medical School. "Black Cohosh May Alter Cell Response to Cancer Therapeutic Agents." *Breast Cancer Research and Treatment.* Apr 2005.

Shahidi, F., Miraliakbari, H. "Evening primrose (Oenothera biennis)." *Encyclopedia of Dietary Supplements.* 2005.

Shell, J.A. "Evidence-based practice for symptom management in adults with cancer: sexual dysfunction." *Oncology Nursing Forum*. 2002.

Shu, Xiao Ou, et al. "The Effects of Green Tea and Exercise in the Reduction of Depression." *J Clin Oncol*. Online; Jan 4, 2010.

Society of Obstetricians and Gynecologists of Canada. "SOGC clinical practice guidelines. The detection and management of vaginal atrophy." *Int J Gynaecol Obstet*. 2005.

Stearns, V., Johnson, M.D., Rae, J.M., Morocho, A., Novielli, A., Bhargava, P., Hayes, D.F., Desta, Z., Flockhart, D.A. "Active tamoxifen metabolite plasma concentrations after coadministration of tamoxifen and the selective serotonin reuptake inhibitor paroxetine." *J Natl Cancer Inst*. 2003.

Suckling, J., Lethaby, A., Kennedy, R. "Local oestrogen for vaginal atrophy in postmenopausal women." *Cochrane Database Syst Rev*. 2003.

Thompson, L.U., Chen, J.M., Li, T., Strasser-Weippl, K., Goss, P.E. "Dietary flaxseed alters tumor biological markers in postmenopausal breast cancer." *Clin Cancer Res*. 2005.

Van der Laak, J.A., de Bie, L.M., de Leeuw, H., et al. "The effect of Replens on vaginal cytology in the treatment of postmenopausal atrophy: Cytomorphology versus computerised cytometry." *J Clin Pathol*. 2002.

Wang, L., Chen, J., Thompson, L.U. "The inhibitory effect of flaxseed on the growth and metastasis of estrogen receptor negative human breast cancer xenograftsis attributed to both its lignan and oil components." *Int J Cancer*. Sep 20, 2005.

Wu, J.P., Fielding, S.L., Fiscella, K. "The effect of polycarbophil gel (Replens) on bacterial vaginosis: A pilot study." *Eur J Obstet Gynecol Reprod Biol*. 2007.

Zhou, S., Xue, C.C., Yu, X., Li, C., Wang, G. "Clinically Important Drug Interactions Potentially Involving Mechanism-based Inhibition of Cytochrome P450 3A4 and the Role of Therapeutic Drug Monitoring." *Therapeutic Drug Monitoring*. Dec 2007; Vol 29, Iss 6.

Ziaei, S., Kazemnejad, A., Zareai, M. "The effect of vitamin E on hot flashes in menopausal women." *Gynecol Obstet Invest*. 2007.

Chapter 9

Dow, K.H. "Having children after breast cancer." *Cancer Practice*. 1994; 2: 407-413.

Hill, W., Fisher, H., Lateiner, D. "The Science of Kissing." *American Association for the Advancement of Science*. Oct 2009.

Largillier, R., Savignoni, A., Gligorov, J., Chollet, P., Guillaume, M., Spielmann, M., Luporsi, E., Asselain, B., Coudert, B., Namer, M. "The effect of pregnancy on the subsequent risk of recurrences after treatment for breast carcinoma." *J Clin Oncol.* 2006; ASCO Annual Meeting Proceedings Part I. Vol 24, No 18S, Abstract No: 553.

Lee, S. J., Schover, L.R., Partridge, A.H., Patrizio, P., Wallace, W.H., Hagerty, K., Beck, L.N., Brennan, L.V., Oktay, K. "ASCO Recommendations on Fertility Preservation in Cancer Patients." *J Clin Oncol.* Jun 20, 2006.

Oktay, K. H., Libertella, N., Buyuk, E., Lostritto, K., Vickers, A., Akar, M. "Letrozole and tamoxifen as safer ovarian stimulants in women undergoing embryo cryopreservation for fertility preservation before breast cancer chemotherapy: A prospective controlled trial." *Am Soc Clin Oncol.* 2005; Abstract No: 539.

Rosen, A. "Third Party Reproduction and Adoption in Cancer Patients." *JNCI Monographs.* 2005.

Chapter 13

Dezentje, V.O., Guchelaar, H.J., Nortier, J.W.R., van de Velde, C.J.H., Gelderblom, H. "Clinical Implications of CYP2D6 Genotyping in Tamoxifen Treatment for Breast Cancer."
Clin. Cancer Res. Jan 2009.

Henry, N.L., Stearns, V., Flockhart, D.A., Hayes, D.F., Riba, M. "Drug Interactions and Pharmacogenomics in the Treatment of Breast Cancer and Depression." *Am J Psychiatry.* Oct 2008.

Perlis, R.H., Fava, M., Neirenberg, A.A., Pollack, M.H., Falk, W.E., Kienke, A.S., Rosenbaum, J.F. "Strategies for Treatment of SSRI-Associated Sexual Dysfunction: A Survey of an Academic Pyschophamacology Practice." *Harvard Review of Psychiatry.* 2002; Vol 10, No 2.

Segraves, R.T., Clayton, A., Croft, H., Wolf, A., Warnock, J.M. "Bupropion Sustained Release for the Treatment of Hypoactive Sexual Desire Disorder in Premenopausal Women." *Journal of Clinical Psychophamacology.* Jun 2004; Vol 24: 3.

Shepherd, J.E. "Therapeutic Options in Female Sexual Dysfunction." *Journal of the American Pharmaceutical Association.* May–Jun 2002; Vol 42: 3.

$\mathscr{I}$ndex

WHAT YOU MUST KNOW ABOUT VITAMINS, MINERALS, HERBS & MORE
Choosing the Nutrients That Are Right for You

Pamela Wartian Smith, MD, MPH

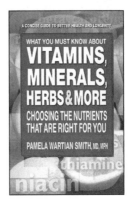

Almost 75 percent of your health and life expectancy is based on lifestyle, environment, and nutrition. Yet even if you follow a healthful diet, you are probably not getting all the nutrients you need to prevent disease. In *What You Must Know About Vitamins, Minerals, Herbs & More,* Dr. Pamela Smith explains how you can restore and maintain health through the wise use of nutrients.

Part One of this easy-to-use guide discusses the individual nutrients necessary for good health. Part Two offers personalized nutritional programs for people with a wide variety of health concerns. People without prior medical problems can look to Part Three for their supplementation plans. If you want to maintain good health or you are trying to overcome a medical condition, *What You Must Know About Vitamins, Minerals, Herbs & More* can help you make the best choices.

$15.95 US • 448 pages • 6 x 9-inch quality paperback • ISBN 978-0-7570-0233-5

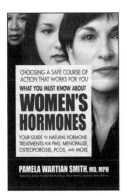

WHAT YOU MUST KNOW ABOUT WOMEN'S HORMONES
Your Guide to Natural Hormone Treatments for PMS, Menopause, Osteoporosis, PCOS, and More
Pamela Wartian Smith, MD, MPH

Hormonal imbalances can occur at any age and for a variety of reasons. While most hormone-related problems are associated with menopause, fluctuating hormonal levels can also cause a variety of other conditions. *What You Must Know About Women's Hormones* is a clear guide to the treatment of hormonal irregularities without the health risks associated with standard hormone replacement therapy.

This book is divided into three parts. Part I describes the body's own hormones, looking at their functions and the problems that can occur if these hormones are not at optimal levels. Part II focuses on the most common problems that arise from hormonal imbalances, such as PMS, hot flashes, and endometriosis. Lastly, Part III details hormone replacement therapy, focusing on the difference between natural and synthetic hormone treatments.

$17.95 US • 256 pages • 6 x 9-inch quality paperback • ISBN 978-0-7570-0307-3

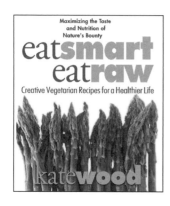

EAT SMART EAT RAW
Creative Vegetarian Recipes for a Healthier Life
Kate Wood

From healing diseases to detoxifying your body, from lowering cholesterol to eliminating excess weight, the many important health benefits derived from a raw vegetarian diet are too important to ignore. However, now there is another compelling reason to go raw—taste! In her new book *Eat Smart, Eat Raw,* cook and health writer Kate Wood not only explains how to get started, but also provides delicious kitchen-tested recipes guaranteed to surprise and delight even the fussiest of eaters.

Eat Smart, Eat Raw begins by explaining the basics of cooking without heat, from choosing the best equipment to stocking your pantry. What follows are twelve recipe chapters filled with truly exceptional dishes, including hearty breakfasts, savory soups, satisfying entrées, and luscious desserts.

$15.95 US • 184 pages • 7.5 x 9-inch quality paperback • ISBN 978-0-7570-0261-8

THE WORLD GOES RAW COOKBOOK
An International Collection of Raw Vegetarian Recipes
Lisa Mann

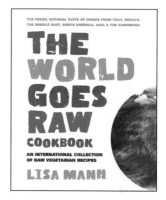

People everywhere know that meals prepared without heat can taste great and improve their overall health. Yet raw cuisine cookbooks have always offered little variety—until now. In *The World Goes Raw Cookbook,* raw food chef Lisa Mann provides a fresh approach to (un)cooking with recipes that have an international twist.

After discussing the healthfulness of a raw food diet, *The World Goes Raw Cookbook* tells you how to stock your kitchen with the tools and ingredients that make it easy to prepare raw meals. What follows are six recipe chapters, each focused on a different ethnic cuisine, including Italian, Mexican, Middle Eastern, Asian, Caribbean, and South American dishes. And from soups and starters to desserts, every one's a winner. There are even easy-to-follow instructions for growing fresh ingredients in your own kitchen garden.

Whether you are already interested in raw food or are exploring it for the first time, the taste-tempting recipes in *The World Goes Raw* can add delicious variety to your life.

$16.95 US • 194 pages • 7.5 x 9-inch quality paperback • ISBN 978-0-7570-0320-2

THE DŌ-IN WAY
Gentle Exercises to Liberate the Body, Mind, and Spirit
Michio Kushi

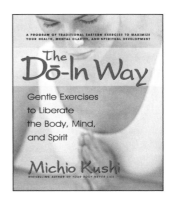

Dō-In is an ancient traditional exercise for the cultivation of physical health, mental serenity, and spirituality. Over the last 5,000 years, it has served as the origin of such well-known disciplines as shiatsu, acupuncture, moxibustion, yogic exercises, and meditation. Literally meaning to pull and stretch, Dō-In originated as a way of achieving longevity and attaining the highest potential of mental and spiritual development.

Dō-In techniques are a series of successive motions designed to harmonize body systems. *The Dō-In Way* details the fundamental aspects of this exercise, which involves breathing, posture, and self-massage and manipulation to stimulate body systems. The gentle application of pressure on the body's meridians corresponds directly with physical processes, and allows for the conditioning and stimulation of internal organs. This is a comprehensive handbook to an ancient system of movement designed to enhance physical, mental, and spiritual health.

$15.95 US • 224 pages • 7.5 x 9-inch quality paperback • ISBN 978-0-7570-0268-7

BIG YOGA
A Simple Guide for Bigger Bodies
Meera Patricia Kerr

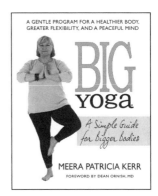

If you think yoga is only for skinny young things, you need to think again. To expert Meera Patricia Kerr, yoga can and should be used by everyone—*especially* plus-size individuals. In her new book, *Big Yoga,* Meera shares the unique yoga program she developed for all those who think that yoga is not for them.

Part One of *Big Yoga* begins with a clear explanation of what yoga is, what benefits it offers, and how it can fit into anyone's life. The book goes on to provide practical information regarding clothing, mats, and suitable environments, and to emphasize the need to begin with care. Part Two offers over forty different exercises specifically designed to work with bigger bodies.

If you have thought that yoga is not for you, pick up *Big Yoga* and let Meera Patricia Kerr help you become more confident and relaxed than you may have ever thought possible.

$17.95 US • 240 pages • 7.5 x 9-inch quality paperback • ISBN 978-0-7570-0215-1

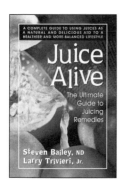

JUICE ALIVE
The Ultimate Guide to Juicing Remedies
Steven Bailey, ND and Larry Trivieri, Jr.

The world of fresh juices offers a powerhouse of antioxidants, vitamins, minerals, and enzymes. The trick is knowing which juices can best serve your needs. In this easy-to-use guide, health experts Dr. Steven Bailey and Larry Trivieri, Jr. tell you everything you need to know to maximize the benefits and tastes of juice.

The book begins with a look at the history of juicing. It then examines the many components that make fresh juice truly good for you—good for weight loss and so much more. Next, it offers practical advice about the types of juices available, as well as buying and storing tips for produce. The second half of the book begins with an important chart that matches up common ailments with the most appropriate juices, followed by over 100 delicious juice recipes. Let *Juice Alive* introduce you to a world bursting with the incomparable tastes and benefits of fresh juice.

$14.95 • 272 pages • 6 x 9-inch quality paperback • ISBN 978-0-7570-0266-3

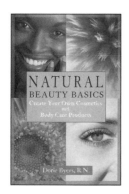

NATURAL BEAUTY BASICS
Create Your Own Cosmetics and Body Care Products
Dorie Byers, RN

Every day, television and magazine ads tell us that beautiful skin and hair are available only through the use of expensive brand-name products. But the fact is that you can attain a radiant, healthy appearance by using products made inexpensively at home. That's what *Natural Beauty Basics* is all about. First, author Dorie Byers guides you to the equipment and ingredients you'll need to make your own products. She then presents easy-to-follow recipes for over 150 hand creams, body powders, shampoos, soaps, and more—products that are effective, all-natural, and allergen-free.

You don't have to spend a lot of money to get the best possible care for your hair, skin, and nails. Whether you enjoy making your own beauty products at home, you are in search of products that are allergen- and chemical-free, or you simply love to pamper yourself, your first stop should be *Natural Beauty Basics.*

$14.95 • 208 pages • 6 x 9-inch quality paperback • ISBN 978-1-890612-19-1